CW00551130

Physiotherapy in
Veterinary Practice

LIBRARY OF VETERINARY PRACTICE

LIBRARY OF VETERINARY PRACTICE

Physiotherapy in Veterinary Practice

MARY W. BROMILEY
MCSP, SRP, RPT (USA)
Chartered Physiotherapist

AIDED BY
BARRY PARK
BVM & S, MRCVS

PATRiCK SWEENEY
MRCVS

Drawings by Penelope Slattery
Photography by Jennifer Slattery
and Tom McQuilton

FOREWORD BY

HRH THE PRINCESS ROYAL

OXFORD

BLACKWELL SCIENTIFIC PUBLICATIONS

LONDON EDINBURGH BOSTON

MELBOURNE PARIS BERLIN VIENNA

Dedicated to the late Sir Charles Strong MCSP, KCVO
The founder of animal physiotherapy

© 1991 by
Blackwell Scientific Publications
Editorial Offices:
Osney Mead, Oxford OX2 oEL
25 John Street, London WC1N 2BL
23 Ainslie Place, Edinburgh EH3 6AJ
3 Cambridge Center, Cambridge,
  Massachusetts 02142, USA
54 University Street, Carlton
  Victoria 3053, Australia

First published 1991

Set by Setrite Typesetters, Hong Kong
Printed and bound in Great Britain at
The Alden Press, Oxford

DISTRIBUTORS
Marston Book Services Ltd
PO Box 87
Oxford OX2 oDT
(*Orders*: Tel: 0865 791155
        Fax: 0865 791927
        Telex: 837515)

USA
  Mosby—Year Book, Inc.
  11830 Westline Industrial Drive
  St Louis, Missouri 63146
  (*Orders*: Tel: 800 633−6699)

Canada
  Mosby—Year Book, Inc.
  5240 Finch Avenue East
  Scarborough, Ontario
  (*Orders*: Tel: (416) 298-1588)

Australia
  Blackwell Scientific Publications
  (Australia) Pty Ltd
  54 University Street
  Carlton, Victoria 3053
  (*Orders*: Tel: (03) 347-0300)

British Library
Cataloguing in Publication Data

Bromiley, Mary W.
  Physiotherapy in veterinary practice.
  1. Veterinary medicine.
  Physiotherapy I. Title   II. Park,
  Barry   III. Sweeney, Patrick
  IV. Series
  636.089582

ISBN 0−632−02833−5

Contents

Foreword by
HRH The Princess Royal

Xenophon advocates 'massage' in his treatise on Horsemanship. Evolution has turned the masseur into the physiotherapist, armed in the final decade of the 20th Century with sophisticated machines to aid healing.

The pioneer of animal physiotherapy was Sir Charles Strong; stationed in Malta before the last war he was asked, by my great uncle, the late Lord Louis Mountbatten, to use his skills to 'repair' injured polo ponies.

Sir Charles continued successfully in the dual role of animal and human physiotherapist until his death; a role in which he treated me and my horses. His advice has guided my own observations and treatment of horses ever since and greatly helped keeping myself fairly fit too.

There is little time for students of veterinary medicine to learn physiotherapy techniques during their training, although the use of such techniques, in aiding the recovery of injured animals, is undeniable.

This book should be of value to vets who wish to use physiotherapy machines to help their patients, and members of the general public who may have purchased or wish to purchase a machine in order to help an animal in their care.

Anne

Preface

Physiotherapy is becoming an accepted treatment within the musculoskeletal section of veterinary medicine. Unfortunately, there is no exposure during veterinary training to the uses and effects of physiotherapeutic equipment. This book will describe the commonly used machines, discuss the effects of these machines on tissues and suggest which, in the authors' opinions, have been of most benefit in a series of named conditions.

It is unfortunate that clients expect 'machine miracles', particularly as most available literature describes accelerated healing. Tissue heals at a predetermined rate; all the machines can do is enhance the ability of tissue to heal. This can only be achieved if the correct machine is correctly applied at the appropriate time. Complete recovery will never be achieved with the machines alone. Active rehabilitation in the form of controlled exercise should go hand-in-hand with the use of machines.

The Veterinary Surgery (Exemptions) Order 1962, permits 'Physiotherapy' as a treatment for animals providing it is carried out at the direction of a registered veterinary surgeon who has examined the animal and prescribed such treatment. There is a specialist group, the Association of Chartered Physiotherapists in Animal Therapy (ACPAT), controlled by the Chartered Society of Physiotherapy, whose members have worked for at least 2 years in the human field and have also seen practice with two veterinary surgeons.

The physiotherapist must work with the knowledge of the veterinary surgeon in charge of the case, who should have provided a diagnosis and prescribed physiotherapy. The physiotherapist should be able to choose the treatment regime suitable for the case in question and should report to the veterinary surgeon regularly.

1 / Large Animal Practice

With the greatly increased use of physiotherapy in the human field during the last 20 years, it is surprising that it is still relatively infrequently applied to the equine patient.

This is probably as a result of the naturally conservative equine owner and veterinary surgeon, who in general are suspicious of all innovations, medical or otherwise. The former prefer to follow the methods of time-honoured tradition and the latter prefer to wait until conclusive scientific proof has been documented before adding anything new to their routine treatments.

Whilst it often proves virtually impossible to make scientific evaluations of the efficacy of physiotherapeutic treatment, there is a great deal of empirical evidence to suggest that many of the injuries treated in the human field are pathologically very similar to those in an equine field. Physiotherapy, therefore, has also become an integral part of the treatment regime used within a veterinary practice.

One must not assume that these treatments are only economically viable for use in the valuable competition horse, because animals cost the same to keep whether they are being exercised or resting through injury; thus, any reduction in the recovery time prevents the rapidly escalating costs of an ornament.

This chapter contains a list of some of the conditions to which current physiotherapy techniques may be applied in order that the recovery time may be shortened and/or the resolution of the lesions be more complete, thus reducing the likelihood of any recurrence of the condition or of it becoming chronic.

Before any of these specified techniques are instigated, it is imperative that a diagnosis is obtained from a veterinary surgeon and that the physiotherapist and vet work in close conjunction throughout any treatment.

Conditions of the foot

Bruising
Solar bruising is probably the most common cause of lameness in the equine. The severity of the bruising can vary from relatively

1

minor conditions to that causing frank haemorrhage or even involving the pedal bone, causing a progressive resorption, i.e. thinning and weakening of the bone, to occur. These lesions can be resolved more quickly if an increased blood supply to the area can be effected.

This has traditionally been achieved by cold hosing and/or hot poulticing. Whilst the basis of the treatment remains the same, use of the 'jacuzzi welly boots' and electrotherapy has increased the efficiency of such treatment. The boot combines low temperature, reduced pressure and a massaging effect to the limb, all of which contribute to an increase in blood flow.

Swimming is a useful aid in any weight-bearing lameness in the fit horse, as loss of muscle tone, or indeed muscle wastage in the more chronic conditions, can be avoided without exacerbating the lameness.

Laminitis
The use of pulsed electrotherapy by applying large electrode pads to the heel area of affected limbs twice daily for 2 hours each treatment has been shown to abbreviate the acute inflammatory process, help in the reduction of pain and allow a prompt return to the normal gait [1].

Sidebone
The use of ultrasound in the acute phase of this condition promotes healing with less bone formation in the lateral cartilages than would be the case with traditional treatments, i.e. using anti-inflammatory and pain-killing drugs.

Fracture of the pedal bone
Use of the magnetic field therapy in the treatment of many types and sites of fractures has been reviewed by Aver, Burch and Hall [2]. They showed that in addition to speeding up bone healing through stimulation of various cellular mechanisms, a pulsing electromagnetic field blocks the inhibiting effect of the parathyroid hormone in collagen synthesis.

They also demonstrated the successful use of this therapy in non-union fractures.

This type of treatment can obviously be used on fractures at many sites in the horse; however, the correct application of the pads at each site is essential and is discussed fully in Chapter 5.

Conditions of the fetlock

Damage to this joint has a great variety of causes, e.g. over extension, concussion, an inco-ordinated stride or even bad conformation.

Damage to the joint surfaces most commonly results in articular windgalls. These are distentions of the joint capsule which appear as swellings between the posterior border of the cannon and the branches of the suspensory ligament (see Fig. 1.1(b)).

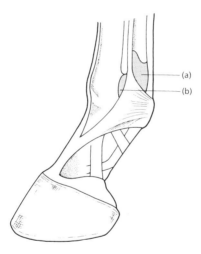

Fig. 1.1 (a) The digital sheath; and (b) the palmar pouch of the fetlock joint capsule.

Physiotherapeutic aids used in these conditions are aimed at reducing inflammation within the joint and thus producing a reduction in the size or tension of the windgalls.

These clinical signs provide an excellent example of the need for a correct diagnosis before any treatment regime is instigated. Fractures of the pastern or lower cannon usually involve the surface of the fetlock joint and result in the formation of windgalls, but passive flexion or ultrasound therapy would be positively harmful in these cases; possibly even disastrous. If a fracture is not present, then the measures to reduce the inflammation and maintain the pre-trauma range of movement in the joint would include these treatments. Magnetic field therapy (MFT), jacuzzi boots and massage are also of value in cases where there is only soft tissue involved or at least no fractured or chipped bone.

As the sesamoid bones are involved in the articulation of the fetlock joint there is often concurrent pathology of their surfaces when trauma to the fetlock joint occurs. This may result in the appearance of tendinous windgalls Fig. 1.1(a), which are a distention of the flexor tendon sheath. They are more commonly seen in hind limbs and are treated in a similar manner to those conditions involving soft tissue damage elsewhere in the fetlock, as described above.

Severe trauma to the joint results in damage to the articular surfaces leading to degenerative arthritic joint disease. Ultrasound and MFT have been found to be effective in the treatment of such conditions. It was found that animals treated with PEM were able to return to full exercise sooner than those with similar conditions using conventional treatments [3].

Conditions of the shins
Sore or 'bucked shins' are most commonly seen in the forelimbs of immature animals stressed by exercise.

The condition is caused by microfractures resulting in irritation of the periosteum and the formation of new bone. Whilst rest is paramount to enable resolution of the condition, MFT, cold laser and jacuzzi boots are used to minimize the irritation and thus reduce the amount of new bone growth. Note that as the condition may involve fractures the use of ultrasound is contraindicated.

As the condition usually occurs in animals required to return to work as soon as possible, swimming is an essential adjuvant to these other treatments in order to maintain muscle tone without the limbs bearing weight.

Splints
These are new bone growths caused by an irritation of the periosteum through stress on the fibrous interosseous ligament between the splint bone and adjacent surface of the cannon. The irritation can also be caused by a blow to the area, usually from the opposing foot.

Treatment in the acute phase aims to disperse inflammatory exudates and haemorrhage and minimize new bone formation. MFT and cold laser are the treatments of choice. Fractures of the splint bone are common, hence the use of ultrasound should be avoided.

Conditions of the knees

Direct trauma caused by falling onto a hard or rough surface can cause a variety of injuries ranging from mild subcutaneous bruising to lacerations and extensive tissue loss, exposing the bone surfaces.

Bruising has been dealt with previously under conditions of the foot (p. 1). However, lacerations provide additional problems of possible infection and exuberant granulation tissue (proud flesh). Cold laser treatment has been suggested as an adjuvant to antibiotics in order to control surface infections. Ultrasound is suggested as an aid to control proud flesh formation, thus allowing new skin to cover the defect as quickly as possible.

Passive flexion of the joint during healing is a necessary procedure in order to maintain full mobility of the joint by gently breaking down fibrous adhesions between tissues before they can become established as scar tissue with the inevitable loss of elasticity in the area.

Inflammatory conditions of the knee capsule and/or bone surfaces are very common because, in progressively faster paces, there is an associated progressive hyperextension of the joint causing abnormal stresses on the bone surfaces and strains on the joint capsule attachments.

It is important to X-ray the joint to ascertain that no fractures are present before using ultrasonic therapy, but MFT or ultrasound can be used to reduce inflammation and maintain full movement in the joint.

Post-operative care after the surgical removal of bone chips or internal fixation of larger fragments should include cold laser therapy to promote healing, along with massage and passive flexion to minimize adhesions.

Conditions of the hocks

Bog spavin
This is a distension of the hock joint capsule and, as stated with previous capsular conditions, cold laser, ultrasound and MFT are useful. This condition often is the result of poor conformation of the hind limbs and may recur despite intensive therapy.

Bone spavin
This is an osteoarthritic condition of the hock joint, hence ultrasound is once again contraindicated but MFT and cold laser in the acute phases can be beneficial.

Thoroughpin
This is a distention of the deep digital flexor tendon sheath where it runs over the hock region. Ultrasound and MFT are useful in reducing the swelling.

Curbs
Curbs are caused by tearing of the calcaneo-metatarsal ligament on the posterior aspect of the hock. In the acute phase the inflammatory reaction can be reduced by the use of cold laser, ultrasound or MFT. Prompt treatment often results in a much smaller blemish than if the condition is left untreated initially.

Conditions of the stifle
The most common cause of injury to this joint is the upward fixation of the patella causing the joint to lock. This presents a classical clinical picture of an animal with a rigidly straight hind limb usually pointing backwards.

The condition is associated with recent loss of condition or irregular exercise. Reduction of the inflammation in the joint is beneficial in the short-term using PEM, cold laser or ultrasound. In order to minimize the chances of recurrence, treatment to strengthen the muscle groups involved in the joint function is essential. Electrical muscle stimulation is the most effective treatment I have used.

Conditions of the tendons and the ligaments
The most common injury to these structures is to the superficial digital flexor tendon of the forelimb. This injury, however mild it may appear initially, should always be treated as an emergency. Immediate first aid measures should include a support bandage from below the knee to the coronary band. The sooner such support can be applied the sooner haemorrhage and inflammatory exudation can be stopped, thus preventing further disruption. The less fluid accumulates within the tendons and their associated sheaths, the less adhesions and permanent scar tissue will be left when the area has healed.

It is in these injuries that ultrasound, magnetic field therapy and cold lasers have been extensively used in order to augment the use of the pressure bandaging. References [4] and [5] chronicle the use of magnetic field therapy in over 200 cases of this type of injury in the lower limb of horses and 170 where cold laser therapy has been used on similar conditions.

If the injury is of such severity that the limb requires casting, then magnetic field therapy (MFT) must be used as it is the only means of treatment that will penetrate a cast.

Recent work at Glasgow University (pers. commun.) appears to indicate that the use of cold laser on these tendons improves the rate of healing during the first 3 or 4 months after injury. The lesions were monitored using ultrasound scanning and compared with a group of untreated, similar injuries.

Electrical muscle stimulation of the tendon's parent muscles may be used to maintain muscle strength in the affected limb. Damage to suspensory or check ligaments should be treated in a similar fashion to that described for tendons, whether they occur separately or in association with them.

Flexor tendon laxity
This condition occurs in newborn foals to varying degrees. The most severe cases can only walk on the posterior aspect of their fetlocks. Therapy aims to prevent trauma to these areas, whilst encouraging flexor effort. Swimming has been advocated for severe cases and affected foals swim well with supervision. This has proved to be a successful method of restoring tone to the flexor musculature [6].

Conditions of the muscles
Bruised or pulled muscles occur for many reasons and in a variety of sites in the horse, from poll to rump. Once a veterinary surgeon has diagnosed the condition as involving soft tissue only, treatment should initially attempt to reduce the bruising or haematoma present and then prevent the development of adhesions as the damaged tissues heal.

Unfortunately muscle damage, if left untreated, often heals with excessive fibrous scarring. This creates a region of reduced elasticity within the muscle, leaving it more prone to a recurrence of a similar injury in that area when the animal is returned to full work.

Cold-water treatment of the affected muscle in the acute phase is very useful, followed by cold laser, ultrasound or interferential therapy, depending on the site and depth of the damaged muscle (see Chapters 7, 8 and 9).

At later stages of healing, electrical stimulation of the affected muscle groups combined with controlled exercise should be used to maintain the muscle efficiency and keep the development of adhesions down to a minimum.

Muscle wastage

This occurs, to some degree, as a sequel in any lameness but is usually more apparent in the very severe or long-standing cases. Electrical stimulation of the affected muscles is essential. Controlled exercise using weights on the limb can be used in conjunction, in order to restore the muscle strength to its original capacity as quickly as possible.

Thoraco-lumbar and pelvic injuries

One of the most frequent diagnoses made by horse owners is that their animal is suffering from a bad back. Many of these cases are subsequently diagnosed by veterinary surgeons as conditions un-related to back pain.

The causes and pathology of most of the conditions affecting the thoraco-lumbar muscles and ligamentous attachments to the spinal column are poorly understood. Whilst spontaneous recovery may occasionally occur due to the release of muscle spasm, the claims that displaced vertebrae in the back can be manipulated is con-sidered implausible by most veterinary practitioners.

Genuine cases of pulled muscles over the thoraco-lumbar and pelvic area obviously do occur. However, due to the depth and mass of muscles involved it is often impossible to locate the exact site of the injury.

Post-mortem work carried out in a survey in South Africa sug-gests that there are many injuries deep in the sacro-iliac region which go undiagnosed throughout a horse's athletic career. This probably accounts for some of the hind limb lameness or the loss of mobility that is never satisfactorily diagnosed. Initial treatments are similar to those for muscle damage in any location, as previously described.

Caution is advised in the use of swimming in the early stages of many of these cases as it may well be contraindicated.

Studies in Queensland Veterinary School have shown that manipulative techniques have some value in the relief of pain due to muscle spasm and possibly in conditions involving the attachments of the first cervical vetebrae. However, it seems likely that muscle spasm is secondary to some other injury and that back pain may well be a combination of two or more conditions.

Wounds

Cold laser therapy has been widely used to increase the rate of wound healing. In studies of 264 wounds of all sizes, including burns, treated between 4 and 6 times each, all showed a good to excellent response to laser treatment [7].

Pain relief after treatment of these cases was significant, due to an alteration in the synthesis of prostaglandins. The increased healing rate is the result of a stimulus of the immune system which greatly reduces the development of any surface infection.

Abscesses and haematomas

Ultrasonic treatment of these conditions causes less organization of the necrotic fluid or blood clot and better differentiation of the liquid from the surrounding tissues. Consequently, when the lesions are opened, better drainage is achieved through a smaller incision and less massage is required to expel any remaining debris.

In conclusion, my experience of the use of physiotherapy in the horse under veterinary supervision has been largely rewarding, even though the exact mode of action of some techniques may not yet be fully understood.

References to Chapter 1

1 Vasko KA, Spauchus A, Lowery M (1986) *Equine Practic*; **8**(4): 28
2 Auer JA, Burch GE, Hall P (1983) Review of pulsing electromagnetic field therapy and its possible application to horses. *Equine Veterinary Journal*, **15**(4): 354−360
3 Focke H, Oldenberg (1981) *Sport and Fed*; **4**(5): 18
4 (1986) *Journal of Equine Medicine & Surgery for the Practitioner*; **8**(2): 24
5 Janes WE (1983) *Equine Veterinary Data*; **4**(22): 337
6 Leitch M (1985) Musculo skeletal disorders in neonatal foals. *Veterinary Clinics of North America*, **1**(1): 198
7 (1986) *Journal of Equine Medicine & Surgery for the Practitioner*; **8**(2): 24

2 / Physiotherapy in Athletic Dogs

Indications for physiotherapy

There is unfortunately some scepticism about the merit of physiotherapy because many patients do not respond to it. Like other therapies, it has its limitations, but disappointing results can often be attributed to one of two factors; it is tried for conditions that are hopeless or for those wrongly diagnosed by unqualified persons. There are many people at large with magical hands or machines, claiming to be able to put back discs, hips or shoulders that are 'out' and muscles or nerves that are 'twisted'. Demand for their services arises from the failure of many serious injuries in horses and hounds to respond to conventional veterinary medicine and surgery. Consequently any owner longing for a cure may become desperate enough to seek the services of someone who is reported, in the racing press, to have put a hand on the winner of a race.

There was also an illusion among the public that the veterinary profession was disinterested in physiotherapy because of its omission from the curricula of our training and because we were not allowed to advertise what it can do. Over recent years there has been notable progress and scientific advances and sophisticated technology has enabled us to give real benefit, not just to the horse, but to many other species. Research into every method by which pain might be alleviated, and publishing our findings, is our ongoing priority.

Veterinary surgeons welcome the recent legislation by the RCVS to allow physiotherapists to treat animals under our direction. These people fully deserved the status conferred on them by the medical profession. They have proved indispensible to all our hospital orthopaedic departments. Animals can derive equal benefit from the assistance that veterinarians look forward to receiving from physiotherapists. The arrangement must also give animal owners more confidence in physiotherapy and may wean some of them away from consulting practitioners of those branches of alternative medicine whose principles are not validated by scientific assessment.

The qualified physiotherapist understands how forces like

acceleration, shock, jerking and friction may adversely affect the locomotion of the athlete, and in treating resultant lameness can advise on prevention of recurrence.

The practice of physical medicine may be defined as consideration and therapy of functional or mechanical faults to complement therapy of any pathological changes discovered after veterinary examination of the animal. Consequently, before relating the forms of physiotherapy I have used, it would seem appropriate to consider the factors which predispose to trauma and enable us to diagnose the cause of poor performance.

While coursing, racing or during training hounds may sustain injury to any part of the locomotor system: bone, joint, ligament, muscle, tendon or nerve. Since the force on the first five of these tissues is influenced by speed and weight, most lameness is seen in big fast dogs. Statistics also show a similarity between the incidence in the large slow specimens and that in smaller and faster types.

The musculoskeletal system of the hound is well adapted for absorbing the normal concussion and stress of the gallop if the following four requisites are considered.

1 Fit and not fatigued.
2 Running over a straight course.
3 On a reasonably level surface.
4 A surface which is yielding, yet dry enough to allow the claws to grip, and not so moist as to allow the claws to skid or to impact so deeply that protraction is hindered.

In ignoring any of these, there is a real risk of exceeding the safe biomechanical load. It is not practical to observe the second requisite, as there is minimal promotion of racing on a straight course. This would allow equal weight distribution on each forelimb, and on each hindlimb, and also equality in the braking, axial and propelling forces exerted.

Racing is primarily organized to provide a medium for gambling. It is staged around curves whose radii are so small that hounds, if they are to maintain momentum in negotiating the 'left-about-turns', must lean at an angle of as much as 40°. In this bizarre posture, quite abnormal dynamic forces are imposed directly on the limbs and indirectly on the spine.

Centrifugal force on curves
When forced to deviate and negotiate a curve a hound must

overcome centrifugal force which would tend to make it fly off on a straight tangential course. For each individual hound this force is inversely proportional to the radius of the curve and is the paramount factor in over-stressing specific areas of the musculo skeletal system on conventional tracks. The more the hound overcomes this force by leaning over, abducting its right paws outside its centre of gravity, and using friction against the surface to enable it to stay close to the inner fence, the more vulnerable it is.

The cancellous tissue in carpal and tarsal bones and in the epiphyses of long bones, though able to absorb the compression from normal loadbearing, may be unable to cope with the additional shearing or cyclical stress. Fracture may result from a single overloading or from too many small loadings too often. This is called 'fatigue fracture'.

Turbulence and uneven pressure on joint surfaces often leads to proteoglycan loss; synovial fluid loses its viscosity and thus fails to provide the lubrication adequate to protect cartilage from erosion or microfracture. Skeletal trauma may be said to result from the stress of a horizontal force being superimposed on the natural vertical force. Safe absorption of force at impact also demands precise timing of the stride and extension and flexion of joints by co-ordinated action of the reciprocal muscles. Acute turns impel fast hounds to adopt the asynchronous action which results in a high incidence of torn muscles and tendons.

It can be argued that whippets, after racing on a straight, are often found to be lame. However, very often they injure themselves in attempting to grasp the lure at the finish.

Any scepticism about the severity of the percussion, while leaning around the anti-clockwise curves, is dispelled by experiencing the horrific toll of injuries in the right carpal and tarsal joints in the adductor muscles of the right thigh and in those toes, metacarpal/tarsal bones and superficial digital flexor tendons nearest to the inner fence on all four limbs.

Careful examination important for diagnosis

Unhurried observation prior to handling hounds is often rewarding and is essential if veterinary practitioners are not to be misled by the adoption of abnormal behaviour or gait in those who are shy or suspicious of strangers. In finding tissue injury, swelling is the most helpful indication and can be quite obvious in greyhounds and in whippets because of their short coats. Familiarity with the conformation of these can enable us to recognize most abnormalities simply by looking at and comparing all the contours on either side of the mid-line. Swelling is less conspicuous in hairy lurchers, deerhounds and salukis and palpation may be necessary for its detection.

In most cases of acute lameness a limb is affected, and observation of the animal as it walks or while it is standing may indicate the site of pain. On the odd occasion when a hound falls while running it may show severe central locomotor dysfunction and trauma to cranial or spinal bones or nerves must be suspected. In both of these situations diagnosis may be confirmed by palpation, thermography, ultrasonography or radiography and appropriate treatment may be commenced without delay. On the other hand, finding the site of mild or chronic discomfort may be difficult even for an experienced veterinary surgeon. Indeed, a thorough examination of a hound with the motivation to chase, in good condition, without any sign of abnormality, but presented because of loss of performance, can demand much time and patience and without seeing it gallop a definite diagnosis may not be possible.

If no swelling is found and there is no gait abnormality at the walk, the possibility of some malfunction of the most vital part of the skeleton must be considered. This is the axis upon which the limbs act to produce all movement.

The spine of the working hound has remarkable flexibility which allows for a great length of stride. It is capable of much more movement than that of any horse and its efficiency is surpassed only by the spine of the big cats. It becomes completely straightened by neuromuscular action at propulsion. The hip joints of hounds also permit a great range of movement; the hind limbs are loosely attached and towards the end of suspension, the marked arching of the spine allows them to be thrust forward to impact well in front of the fore-limbs.

Pelvic injury from propulsive force

Research by Gunn (1978, 1979, 1981) and by Guy and Snow (1981) on the semitendinosus of greyhounds and of other breeds like collies, afghans, labradors, danes and cross-breds showed that muscles of greyhounds had more large fibres, a higher proportion of fast-twitch fibres, and a greater energy production capacity per unit weight of muscle. All of these factors contribute to the work or force produced and in relation to two individuals of equal weight, condition and motivation it can be said that the one with the greater muscular 'capacity' will be capable of greater acceleration and will also be at greater risk of serious injury when stride symmetry is interrupted.

As propulsion is derived from extension of the hind-limbs completely behind the body, through the powerful action of the spinal and femoral muscles, consideration of the force generated through the pelvis is helpful in understanding problems that may arise along the spine. As the pelvic girdle articulates with the horizontal sacrum at an angle of about 30°, the direction of the fully extended femur coincides with that of the ilium and there is minimal obstruction to transmission of force from the limbs to the spine.

However, hip lameness from repeated impaction of the femoral head into the acetabulum during turning is not uncommon. Usually, the pain results from inflammation of the synovial membrane, and provided the hound is rested before degenerative changes affect the cartilage, recovery can be expected. On the rare occasions the acetabulum is fractured, it has nearly always occurred at the start or during the first few strides. The cause may be, that since the limb is not yet fully extended, an excessive amount of force is transmitted vertically to the acetabulum.

Strain of the vertebral column
The thickness of the shock-absorbing discs accounts for about 15% of the total length of the spinal column and provides resistance to compression by the normal extension and flexion demanded by the arching phase of each stride. The pairs of synovial joints between the processes of contiguous vertebrae prevent excessive lateral or rotary movement and much of the backache pain attributed to 'slipped discs' originates from strain of these little joints.

In turning, the vertebral column is subjected to violent stresses, particularly at, or near the cervico-thoracic, thoraco-lumbar and lumbo-sacral joints. Except when the hound has crash-landed, trauma is rarely so severe as to result in a fracture or in luxation of sufficient degree for misalignment of a spinous process to be palpable. But, if during a clinical examination of a patient who is not psychologically disturbed or upset, it is possible to obtain a reaction from gentle palpation or pressure over the back, it can be concluded that there is, at the least, strain of some underlying joint.

Paravertebral pain and spasm
Experience helps in pinpointing the site of the tension, but it can never be categoric. Contrary to faith in the dexterity of chiropractors neither these joints or their components can be moved or manipulated (other than in whelps) nor can any of the abnormalities be seen that enable damage to be defined in a superficial joint such as an interphalangeal. Over-stretching of the ligaments which bind this joint in man or dog can be quite painful, but there is no comparison with the degree of disturbance that may result from a similar insult to any joint of such a dynamic structure as the spine.

The sequel to any twist or rotation of a vertebrum such as the seventh lumbar, must be some inflammation to the lumbosacral joint and to the joint between L6 and L7. Torsion of one of the four intervertebral foramina may cause pressure on an emerging nerve root and the pain may result in spasm in the multifidus, interspinales and intertransversarii muscles. Rotation of the articular processes of L7 will relax the facet joints on one side of it, cause compression of those on the opposite side of the bone and there may be synovitis and capsulitis. The initial mechanical syndrome thus becomes a pathological and physiological dysfunction.

From this summary of the stresses on the locomotor system and the fact that 10 000 greyhounds are discarded from British tracks annually, many of them before they are 2 years old, the demands and necessity for physiotherapy are obvious.

For all patients with acute injuries a period of rest is essential to allow healing to take place. Physiotherapy may hasten the healing process.

Inactivity over more than 10 days causes a proportionate loss in physical fitness. A rational period for rehabilitation must follow to restore the loss before maximum performance should be demanded again. Physiotherapy can constitute a major role in any restorative programme.

There are may methods of applying physiotherapy. Some of the simpler forms are as old as medicine itself and many of them retain their popularity, particularly among experienced practitioners.

Over recent years however, the public have become more impressed by the variety of sophisticated machines produced by modern technology and claimed to have far wider therapeutic possibilities.

Physical therapy of the strained limb-joint

Action of the muscles which cross synovial joints may permit extension, flexion, adduction, abduction, circumduction, rotation, pronation, and supination and the efficiency of such sophisticated function is related to the animal's condition. The ligaments attached to the epiphyses get some support from the proximity of the muscles in maintaining the integrity of joints, but strenuous exercise often disrupts the attachments even in the fit athlete. Joint injury is often found to be the most common cause of lameness in hounds and the prognosis often depends on how soon treatment can be commenced.

Sprain is a vague term commonly used on seeing a hound walking lame and resenting pressure on a joint. The degree of ligamentous damage may be estimated by manipulation. When it is severe, luxation may be obvious from deviation of the distal component. To define the condition fully, X-rays are mandatory and when they reveal no fracture or osseous changes the pain may be due to rupture of the joint capsule and synovitis with release of degradative enzymes or, in hounds who have been running with chronic lameness, to exposure of subchondral bone. It should be remembered that cartilage ulceration will not be revealed until osteophytes have been deposited and another radiograph, after 5 weeks, may determine whether light training may be resumed. Stressful exercise should not be allowed while synovia contains any inflammatory cells or before restoration of its viscosity and hyaluronate content.

Cold therapy

After trauma, periarticular swelling can be expected, and as with other vital tissues like muscle and tendon the control of inflammatory oedema is an urgent consideration. When applied immediately, and maintained for a quarter of an hour, the old ice poultice has a spectacular effect on the effusion and on the pain associated with it.

Over recent years 'Tendon Eze', a gel which retains cold or heat, has been found to be very useful. It looks professional, but may be

no more effective than a plastic bag of something from the re-
frigerator. Similar packs which may be be cooled or warmed are
widely used in human medicine. In treating inflammatory oedema,
cold gel may be used during alternate 30 minutes, on the day of
the injury. On the following day it may be more effective if used
alternately with heated gel so as to cause constriction and dilation
of the blood supply to the area in turn.

Dressings impregnated with calcium alginate, obtained from
seaweed, have recently become popular for drawing exudate from
traumatized or infected tissue. There is nothing new about the
theory of its action; the cold weed itself was used on contaminated
wounds by the healers of ancient times.

Compression therapy

Where subcutaneous haemorrhage is suspected at the site of an
acute injury, a compression bandage over the ice is indicated. After
limb injuries, even to tissue as proximal as the elbow or stifle joint,
it is not uncommon for swelling to involve the entire limb right
down to the toe nails within 24 hours. The value of intermittent
compression in dealing with this alarming complication was
emphasized by Pflug (1975).

Nowadays plastic 'air splints' which can be inflated by mouth are
carried as standard equipment in ambulances for patients with
circulatory impairment or fractures in limbs. Physiotherapists
working in hospitals use garments specially designed to fit different
sizes of arms and legs and inflate them with a pump unit which is
operated by a compressor.

Heat therapy

The practice of applying heat to treat injury and disease probably
began shortly after primitive man learned how to light a fire. Some
of the methods of using it satisfy modern scientific appraisal; others
are considered suspect or contraindicated. The efficacy and the
ethical justification for the ancient practice of 'firing' were recently
investigated at Bristol University and the report by Silver *et al.*
(1982) has ensured that more aesthetic means of treating tendon
injuries are now being pursued.

The principle behind the application of heat is of course quite
sound but, as with cold, intensity and duration must be controlled
in order to avoid damage to the structure or physiology of the
tissues. The aim is to achieve a rise in temperature (up to 4°C),

vasodilation, increased circulation of blood and lymph, improved metabolism through more oxygen and phagocytes becoming available, and reduction in swelling with consequent alleviation of pain so that the patient may rest, be happy and take nourishment. Forms of heat may be supplied or delivered to the tissues by three means.

Conduction. The warm poultice has been used for centuries throughout the world as a means of treating pain and a great many ingredients have proved to be of some benefit. For their hygroscopic action, in drawing pus or slough out of abscesses or infected wounds, common and epsom-salt are still very much in favour although we now use a refined exsiccated form of the latter. The clay that gave relief in bygone days probably contained aluminium silicate and this with boric acid and methyl salicylate is now dispensed as 'cataplasma kaolini'.

A poultice commonly used is a dressing containing bassorin and boric acid and marketed as Animalintex. It can prove invaluable in a variety of inflammatory conditions and has the advantage in that it sets firm and supports fractured bones and luxated joints. Care must be taken against using it too hot especially in white or fawn animals whose skin may be sensitive to it. A simple method of applying heat to areas proximal to the elbows and stifles, where a hot pack cannot be easily bandaged or strapped on, is by fomentation with gamgee tissue or cotton wool which has been immersed in hot water and wrung out.

For chronic inflammation of the musculoskeletal system there is an old remedy called Thermogene. This is really cotton wool impregnated with the rubifacients capsicin and methyl salicylate and seems to provide analgesic as well as thermal effects when applied around joints under a bandage. It can be beneficial in the treatment of lumbago when stitched to the inside of the rug or kennel-coat.

Radiant heat. Since their discovery, infrared rays have been used extensively, not merely in therapy, but to keep animals warm and comfortable in their quarters. They play a vital role in preventing chill in those who have been out for exercise in wet or cold weather. Some feel threatened by the brightness of luminous lamps and are happier under the dull variety which has less penetrative power.

Conversive heat. Research by Tesla and by d'Arsonval around 1890, proved that high frequency electrical oscillations could be produced with safety in living tissues and led to the introduction of diathermy in medicine. Impressed by reports of this more penetrative type of heat in 1952, the author purchased a short wave diathermy machine with an electromagnetic oscillator which generated alternating current through a cable. This, in pancake form, was placed over the muscles of the back, shoulder or thigh, or in coil form over an injured limb. The theory behind the use of the high frequency current was to get physiological effects from the stimulation of the circulation that would result from generation of heat in the deeper tissues. It would not heat the skin or stimulate excitable tissue.

This machine gained popularity with physiotherapists throughout the fifties for animal and human complaints. The somewhat clumsy coils have been replaced by more practical applicators in the modern microprocessor controlled units. These allow for a wide range of pulse frequency for optimum effect on cell metabolism with optional use of the thermal effects from the continuous mode.

Diathermy is used on many hounds with problems like tendonitis, myositis, adhesions, muscle spasm, paravertebral pain and stiffness of joints following immobilization for the treatment of luxation or fracture.

After a few years, assessment of the new heat therapy showed that a higher proportion of patients were fit to perform again, than were achieved in the years before the author acquired the machine.

The importance and success rate of treatment, and indeed with any forms of physiotherapy, would be lower if hounds were admitted with joint degeneration or with major disruption of tendons or muscles. A comfortable kennel and a nourishing diet; as much exercise as is tolerable and daily massage must also be provided.

The importance of all four of these requirements must be emphasized for the resolution of injury and resumption of training. After any significant injury no form of therapy should, on its own, be considered to offer a realistic chance of restoring optimum athletic capacity.

Exercise. In addition to decline in efficiency of the vital cardiovascular and respiratory systems, confinement in excess of 7 days

results in loss of protein and enzymes from muscles, demineraliz-
ation of bone and deficiency in joint cartilage and synovia. A
rational excercise programme of ascending intensity over a period
must follow in order to restore tissue loss and functional strength.

Those so incapacitated that they cannot walk out for more than a
few minutes at least six times a day, require having their joints
manipulated by grasping their paws and flexing and extending the
limbs as vigorously as their disability will allow. When full
manipulation causes no discomfort the weightless exercise in
swimming can help to get invalids ambulant. The novice can be
stressed by the initial immersion and may be less fearful on seeing a
water-loving dog jump in to retrieve a bit of timber.

Walking exercise should commence on turf as the jarring or
dynamic force on weakened limbs is less than when impacting on
the hard road. Happy patients tend to heal better, and since
hounds are animated by the sight of game, walks across fields may
also have a tonic effect. Gradual increase in the tempo improves
cardiopulmonary efficiency. Trotting enhances the levels of oxygen,
enzymes, glycogen, creatine phosphate and adenosine triphosphate
necessary for muscular metabolism, but several short gallops are
essential to develop the capacity for the energy demanded in
coursing or racing.

Massage. This art is considered to be the cardinal requisite for the
successful practice of physiotherapy or the training of any athlete.
When applied with reasonable pressure or kneading, it stimulates
the blood supply to the muscles, thus dispersing waste products.
The latter effect is particularly valuable in the case of fatigued,
damaged or painful muscles in which lactic acid or dead cells have
accumulated. As well as relieving spasm, touch by sympathetic
hands exerts a calming influence on an anxious patient.

The hound to be treated should be secured in a quiet room of
comfortable temperature. The hands of the masseur or masseuse
should be warmed and be lightly smeared with coconut or olive oil.
The operation must begin with light strokes in a slow or unhurried,
deliberate but gentle manner in order to relax the hound. The
pressure and rate of movement over each area should gradually
increase and then level off. A thorough massage demands that each
group of muscles: neck, back, loins, shoulders, thighs, and fore-
and hindlimbs right down to the paws, is treated for not less than 5
minutes. After a week or so the muscles will be seen to stand out

prominently and will have more tone and suppleness.

Electric rotary or vibratory machines may be used provided the entire body surface is first stroked and palpated to detect any tension, particularly on the day following exercise when muscles may be sore because of the presence of lactate and/or hydroxy-proline. It is not necessary to use liniments containing rubifacients prior to the routine massage, but they should be regarded as essential immediately before competing since many muscles are injured simply because they are stressed while they are cold.

Ultrasonotherapy

The interest in the biological effect of ultrasound arose around 1930 after research by Wood and Loomis demonstrated that paramecia disintegrated when insonated by an ultrasound beam. This little organism had already contributed to medical science when Raab, 30 years earlier, showed the cytotoxic effect of visible light on it and thus introduced photodynamic therapy of localized neoplasia.

The findings from the early clinical trials with ultrasound were promising and by 1960 machines were being added to the equipment in orthopaedic departments of hospitals worldwide. There were many reports that the mechanical vibrations from high frequency sound waves offered distinct advantages over the electrical oscillations produced by diathermy.

Like diathermy, ultrasound also produces heat but it was claimed to be more efficient in that its heat is directed straight into affected tissue without warming the surrounding healthy tissue. It has the advantage in that it is absorbed more by muscle than by fat. At lower frequencies it can penetrate more deeply. In addition to its thermal effects, ultrasound causes micromassage. The mechanical reaction causes biochemical changes in the tissues with improvement in blood supply, lymph flow and intracellular metabolism.

Certain precautions should be observed in using this therapy. Heat is cumulative, particularly in bone cortex, and can cause pain and burns. The risk of overheating can be reduced by using pulsed output rather than continuous, and by moving the transducer slowly around in a circle. Another reaction from an excess of insonation is fatigue or even weakness due to depletion of blood sugar and blood cells. When directed at the chest ultrasound may cause cardiac spasm and it can have drastic consequences if aimed at a thrombus or a tumour. Despite the legislation to protect animals, greyhounds are often seen who have been treated with an ultrasonic or other potentially harmful machine by people without knowledge of its action or of canine anatomy or physiology.

After reading the *Textbook for Physiotherapists* by Summer and Patrick (1964) the author tried ultrasound for the conditions he had been treating with diathermy. It was found that the application was more rewarding probably because it was used in the early stage of injuries. A pronounced analgesic effect on bone, post fracture, and on joints with arthritis was found to occur. It also helped in starting resolution in torn muscles.

Muscle has an inherent capacity to heal and the prognosis for minor tears with little haemorrhage is favourable. Studies by Schmallbruch (1976) showed that regeneration takes place by the formation of new cells and by repair of damaged myofibre which grows from healthy tissue back into the necrotic area. The problem with more severe ruptures is that they are usually complicated by extensive haemorrhage. Its control and the resorption of the haematoma to permit apposition of fibres, commencement of the regenerative process and prevention of fibrosis and adhesions are urgently necessary.

There is little success with surgery for repair of muscles with gross fibre separation and none from injections of steroids and sclerosing agents but ultrasound often seemed to be useful, at least in curtailing the inflammatory phase and dispersing the extracellular fluid.

In commencing treatment of torn muscle the sound head should be aimed not at the haematoma, for fear of increasing the haemorrhage, but around it. As swelling subsides, the circles of application may gradually converge towards the centre of the haematoma. With the relief of the pressure on the nerve-endings within the endomysium, pain subsides. Gentle hand-massage may be tolerated and light exercise may be resumed as the maturation phase of the healing process commences. This phase may last for 3 months or longer.

The extent and duration of the haematoma and the amount of adhesions formed during the period of inactivity influence the degree of resultant atrophy. Treatment by ultrasound soon after injury and by electronic neuromuscular stimulation from about a month post trauma helps in controlling atrophy.

Daily stimulation can help in stretching the muscle, breaking down the adhesions and contracting the scar. The diffusion of ions of sodium, potassium and calcium associated with the activation of the actin and myosin filaments may also stimulate capillary proliferation and aid in preparing the muscle to undertake the exercise programme necessary for the restoration of maximum functional capacity.

A variety of devices have been developed to provide sinusoidal, faradic or galvanic current through an electrode placed over the motor end plate. Machines must be programmed to operate at definite frequencies, must allow rest periods for the muscle between contractions and must not cause pain.

Muscles may also be stimulated by the interferential machine which is commonly used in the treatment of sports injury. This therapy, introduced by Dr Nemec in Austria in 1955, involves electrodes being placed so that two alternating currents of differing frequencies are directed to cross over and interact at a specific point in excitable tissue. The low frequency current is said to influence pain reduction and also enhancement of circulation as result of stimulation of the parasympathetic system.

Since stimulation can develop a superficial muscle that is unfit for normal exercise, some trainers think that it is beneficial right up to the day of a race and are unaware that excess or inappropriate use of the current may cause imbalance in the muscles or even degeneration of muscle cells.

Salmons and Verbova (1969) working with rabbits found that stimulation of fast-twitch muscle, at a frequency corresponding to the impulse rate of a motoneuron to a slow-twitch muscle, transforms it into a slow type.

Heilmann and Pette (1980) showed that the change in twitch characteristics resulted from molecular alteration of the sarcoplasmic reticulum of the fast-twitch fibres.

In treating strained ligaments or tendons associated with the phalangeal, carpal or tarsal joints ultrasound is more effective if the limb is immersed in a bath of de-aerated water. As absorption of ultrasound in water is negligible the insonation head may be held in the water, about half an inch from the affected tissue or, against an area of the outer side of the bath, smeared with coupling medium.

Ultrasound is also beneficial for the myopathy commonly seen after severe exercise in hounds that are not fully conditioned. Fit greyhounds and whippets may be stressed after a 1-minute course. Differences in their nervous systems and in the histochemical properties of their limb muscles may enable deerhounds to run for 3 minutes and salukis for 5 minutes before tiring.

Hypoxia, electrolyte imbalance, lactic acid accumulation, lysis of cells and myoglobin release into the urine (myoglobinuria) are usually associated with this syndrome. Intensive medical care is vital as untreated cases may die from renal failure. Survivors may be stiff from painful myositis, especially of the rhomboideus, spinalis, semispinalis and longissimus, with hypersensitive tender areas (trigger points) in the skin over the affected muscles. The period of stiffness is indicative of the degree of fibre degeneration and also the rehabilitation required for the return of athletic capacity.

Pulsed electromagnetic field (PEMF)

Another method of using conversive heat in physiotherapy is by application of a pulsed electromagnetic field (PEMF).

The author's first experience of magnetic field therapy was in 1967 when he saw a simple magnetic foil dressing adhesed to a greyhound at a Portugese coursing meeting. Hearing that the magnetic flux density of the heat-reflective foil was about 700 gauss and that the force could penetrate to about half an inch, he tried it on a number of cases with superficial contusions and strains at, and distal to the level of the carpal and tarsal joints. The author saw no evidence of enhanced healing but thermography showed dermal warming which may have given some benefit.

There has since been much scientific evidence of biological effects such as modification of cell behaviour and enhanced production of collagen and proteoglycan from magnetic fields stimulated by current from a pulse generator to a pair of electric coils. A variety of devices have been marketed for delivery of these energies but because of the dearth of definitive reported results of trials on their clinical use by veterinary surgeons there is much confusion as to how these machines may be used to advantage and a degree of scepticism about the benefit animals may be deriving from them. Therefore it seems appropriate to mention some of the publications which created interest in their therapeutic potential.

This therapy for skeletal problems may be said to stem from the initial experimental work of Bassett and Becker (1962) to produce an osteogenic reaction with magnetic fields. Continuing this pioneer work at Columbia University in New York, Bassett with colleagues Pawluk and Pilla (1974) performed bilateral fibular osteotomies on beagles and then applied low frequency PEMF to one limb of each beagle. After 28 days, tests with a mechanical apparatus for stability followed by histology showed, for the first time, that this therapy could enhance the rate of repair in limbs.

Encouraged by these results (Pawluk & Pilla 1977) PEMF was applied to non-union fractures in humans and the report of their success created much interest among orthopaedic surgeons. Their findings were corroborated by Mulier and Spaas (1980). These surgeons applied low frequency current of 10 volts to 19 patients with non-unions and succeeded in getting functional union with bony bridging over the gap region in 7.

In a survey of 83 patients with ununited fractures over an average period of 1.5 years, Bassett *et al.* (1982) described the use of this therapy following bone grafting. Forty five patients, who had initially been treated unsuccessfully with PEMF alone, had bone-grafting and were re-treated with the current. This time 93% healed. The other 38 were initially treated with grafts and the current and achieved a rate of successful healing of 87%. The average time to union for both groups was 4 months.

Bassett (1982) proposed that different pulses are effective at various stages of repair. One to trigger DNA synthesis during the week after injury; another to stimulate synthesis of collagen and proteoglycan during the second week; and the last to enhance calcification, after callus has been produced.

Failure to recognize these parameters may account for some of the negative results reported on this therapy. If it is to be used efficiently, the optimum pulses must be investigated and every patient carefully monitored. In practice veterinary practitioners are dependent on clinical research for guidance on the use of any new method of treatment and for its evaluation. This must involve comparison of what are thought to be cures against an equal number of controls so as to avoid claims for success after the treatment of self-limiting conditions.

Indications for PEMF in veterinary orthopaedics
After reduction with compression of fragments in uncomplicated fractures in fit hounds, immobilization for 6 weeks usually results in union. When this period of disuse must be extended PEMF may be considered in order to control osteoporosis. It may also be

considered advisable immediately after surgery on aged or poorly nourished dogs whose bones tend to have thin cortices from a reduction in numbers or activity of osteoblasts.

The two coils can be fastened to the plaster cast for 8 to 12 hours daily and must be placed opposite to each other at the level of the fracture site to produce a uniform field in the healing tissue. When a magnetic implant has been inserted it is important to use low intensity of current in order to reduce the risk of corrosion from electrolysis.

X-rays of fractures allowed to remain unstable for some weeks usually reveal incomplete apposition of fragments and persistant fibrocartilage in the gap. As an alternative to a cancellous bone graft in such situations PEMF therapy with bursts of 15 Hz may be sufficient to stimulate calcification.

If an avascular cortical graft is used, complementing it with the current might be considered as Sturmer *et al.* (1985) reported that it enhanced haversian remodelling in cortical bone grafts in dogs. There is evidence that a single pulse of 72 Hz exerts a greater influence on increasing blood supply.

PEMF effect on ligaments
Since the biological effects of many machines manufactured for the demanding task of treating athletic injuries have been demonstrated only in caged rodents, claims for and expectations from them should be moderate. After hearing that a magnetic field device was recommended for ligamentous injury, the author tried it for strained and torn interphalyngeal ligaments. It seemed to have some analgesic effect, probably by reducing the production of pro-staglandin, but in no case did a ligament withstand the stress of galloping.

From the scientific literature available, a report by Frank *et al.* (1983) might be the basis of the claim for the device. Their research did show an increase in collagen after treatment of sutured collateral stifle ligaments of rabbits with electromagnetic stimulation but, after 6 weeks, they found no mechanical property differences between the experimental and control ligaments.

PEMF effect on tendons
As severe athletic exercise always results in the death of some collagen fibres in tendons, some degree of tearing is likely if

the stress is repeated before they have been replaced. Routine application of cold bandages immediately after strenuous exertion is a wise precaution adopted by many trainers and when any sign of inflammation is manifested next morning, after palpation or by ultrasonography, some form of therapy is commenced. Recently magnetopulse devices have become popular because of evidence of their beneficial effects.

Binder *et al.* (1984) reported the use of PEMF for tendonitis in humans and the achievement of marked pain relief. In experiments with electromagnetic fields on injured tendons in dogs, McGillivary and Standish (1984) achieved a strength of 92% of normal against a strength of 49% in control tendons.

Such a result in slow-moving canines would be considered perfectly adequate, but for the cursorial breeds, repair which gives total strength is crucial. After rupture, new collagenous fibres tend to be different from the original type 1. They tend to be less elastic, to be laid down in a random irregular pattern and healed ligamants and tendons (even when allowed 3 months for remodelling), lack the tensile strength of the original tissue.

Laser (amplified coherent monochromatic light) therapy

During the past 10 years there has been more interest in the potential of the laser than in any other instrument used in physiotherapy. Because of confusion among the lay public of the potency of low energy laser light with that of the thermo-coagulant or destructive argon, carbon-dioxide, neodymium and ruby beams used so successfully in surgery, there is a certain amount of blind faith in the therapeutic version for intractable or even incurable conditions.

Therapeutic lasers used in medicine work on very low power and produce no measurable thermal effect. The most common are the helium−neon gas lasers with a continuous beam of visible light on a wavelength of 632.8 nm and infrared lasers with a more penetrating pulsating beam of 904 nm wavelength. There are also machines which incorporate both of these media, some of which may be used in continuous or pulsed mode, some which offer a choice of wavelength through interchangeable probes and still others with a special diagnostic probe which appeal to owners wishing to save on veterinary consultations.

In a variety of cases afflicted with wounds, contusions, cellulitis, neuropathy, myopathy and fibrositis the laser, despite the author's uncertainty about the optimum dosage, frequency or intensity, seemed to have some effect on pain. The facial expression of some hounds was less distressed and they became less aggressive or less apprehensive. After using many painless therapies the influence of a gentle touch and the soothing words of nursing staff on such behavioural changes can not be undervalued. Lasering of some patients may also have helped in the reduction of oedema, resorption of haematoma and fibrin, stimulation of the blood circulation and lymph drainage and enhancement of tissue metabolism. Review of the relevant literature indicates that the whole concept of laser therapy remains controversial and its practice requires further investigation.

Laser radiation of wounds

The late Professor Endre Mester of Budapest became one of the pioneers of laser application to medicine and with colleagues (1968) he showed that it could stimulate wound healing. There is rarely any cause for concern about union of severed healthy skin or other tissue; opposing its edges can be expected to result in union after 10 days but the discovery was considered of major significance for the treatment of those wounds necessitating skin-grafting or involving trauma, loss of blood supply and infection.

Mester et al. (1971) continuing their experiments with the ruby laser, applied it to burns inflicted on the backs of mice by electrocoagulation. They found that radiation at a dose rate of 1 joule per square centimetre twice weekly stimulated healing or increased the rate of healing.

Mester et al. (1983) in publishing the results of their clinical and experimental work on wounds, listed the effects of lasers on different biological systems: prostaglandin production, RNA, DNA and albumin synthesis in fibrocyte cultures, increase in collagenous fibres, phagocytosis of leucocytes, proliferation of new blood vessels and increase in tensile strength of sutured wounds.

These findings were supported by Lievens (1986) after a controlled experiment at the University of Brussels. He used a He−Ne infrared laser on 100 out of 600 rats with abdominal incisions. In the radiated wounds oedema disappeared sooner, there was earlier regeneration of vein and lymph vessels, regeneration of wounds occurred after 7 days as against 14 in the controls and adhesions were very rare.

Extensive research seems to indicate that while in many cases laser therapy will accelerate the initial healing of wounds, there is no increase in the tensile strength of the final scar. Research by Karu (1988) suggests that the photostimulative effect of lasers can initiate cell proliferation in unfavourable conditions of o_2 tension, pH, etc.

As with PEMF therapy, some of the conflicting results with lasers may be due to differences in the amount of energy being delivered to the tissue, or to the use of different pulse frequencies. This effect was demonstrated in experiments with a combined pulsed IR and continuous wave He–Ne laser on mice at Guy's Hospital by Dyson and Young (1986).

These two scientists, in irradiating wounds compared the effects of variation in the infrared pulse frequency. They achieved an increase in wound contraction in the mice treated at a frequency of 700 Hz while inhibition of contraction resulted in those treated at 1200 Hz. In the group treated at 700 Hz there was a higher total cell-count and a higher fibroblast-count; also the fibroblasts were aligned parallel to each other as opposed to being more irregularly arranged in the 1200 Hz recipients.

Lasering of tendons
Since tendon injury is so common and often so serious in athletes, it is probably true that every known therapy has been applied to it. The laser is no exception but there is little clinical evidence that it is a specific remedy.

McKibbin and Paraschak (1983) in Ontario studied the effects of treating chronic bowed tendons in horses with a He–Ne infrared laser with a wavelength of 904 nm. They reported that a significant number returned to racing and gave satisfactory performances. It would have been more informative and complete if it had included an evaluation of the tendons on the day following the stress.

In a double-blind study of using a He–Ne infrared laser on 64 patients with tendinopathy at Munich University Medical School, Siebert *et al.* (1987) concluded that it was not effective. They treated 32 patients with the laser switched on and 32 with it switched off for 15 minutes on 10 consecutive days and achieved an identical result for each group (50% reduction for resting pain, and 30% for movement and pressure pain).

In a controlled study to assess IR laser therapy of shoulder tendonitis in patients at Queen Elizabeth and General Hospitals

Birmingham, England et al. (1989) reported that it reduced pain and facilitated joint movement. They also advocated more studies to decide on optimum frequency and treatment regimens.

The clinical work by Yamada et al. (1989), at Obihiro University in Japan, is worthy of special mention because, as well as being directed at some tendon injuries, it was based on acupuncture and the results may be considered phenomenal. They used a gallium aluminium arsenide diode laser on acupoints in 15 horses and claimed that they cured 6 out of 7 with flexor tendonitis; 3 out of 5 with suspensory desmitis; 1 of 1 with fetlock injury; and 2 of 2 with ejaculation deficiency. In addition to pain suppression, they reported improvement of inflammatory reaction and rapid cures.

Of all the cases listed as 'cured', the most interesting was the racehorse who had a 'bowed' tendon for 3 weeks. It was lasered at 10 mW for 20 to 40 seconds once a day for 7 days on each side of the bowed area. It walked soundly after the second day and the swelling disappeared after the sixth day. It raced and won on the third day after discharge. The report stated that the tendonitis cases remained cured for between 4 days and 3 months. Therefore it seems that this racehorse remained cured on the day after it had raced.

Neurophysiological effects on nerves
In the debate over the value of laser therapy there appears to be less argument over its effect on nerves than on any other tissue. But there is some.

In a double-blind study, Walker (1983) in Los Angeles found that irradiation with a He−Ne laser relieved pain in 19 out of 26 patients who had chronic neuralgia, osteoarthritis, sciatica or neuropathy. Analgesia was observed after exposure of the skin overlying the radial, medial and saphenous nerves or of the appropriate painful nerve and the urine of patients showed an increased excretion of the metabolite of serotonin. Those who received sham stimulation reported no pain relief.

Basford et al. (1987) however, in a controlled study of patients suffering from thumb osteoarthritis, found no difference between those treated with a 0.9 mW He−Ne laser and those for whom the machine was not switched on. Walker and Akhanje (1985) proved that laser irradiation could stimulate peripheral nerves. They applied a He−Ne laser to the wrist over the median nerve and by electrical recordings achieved a propogated response at the shoulder. However, Wu *et al.* (1986) conducted a series of experiments at three separate laboratories in the USA and, although achieving a response by electrical stimulation, they failed to find any evidence of a He−Ne laser-evoked response.

But experiments by Rochkind *et al.* (1987) showed that the He−Ne laser could not only produce nerve stimulation but also regenerate nerve tissue damaged by crush injury in dogs.

Laser treatment in acupuncture
The Chinese, for 3 000 years, have been sticking needles, as fine as 30 gauge, into humans, equines and other animals and twirling them. Despite the lingering mysticism about acupuncture its potential to relieve pain, in some subjects, is generally recognized. Any scepticism that veterinary practitioners have about acupuncture can be dispelled when it is shown that its effects, such as the release of serotonin and endogenous peptides like endorphins and encephalins, were transferred from one animal to another by blood transfer.

Some acupuncturists now inject a few minims of a sterile fluid about once a week, some implant gold or silver beads about once a year and others use transcutaneous electronic nerve stimulators to generate small amplitude pulsed square waves. These stimulate afferent nerves and produce a tingling sensation. Neural effects from electrical stimuli are easily understandable since equipment has been developed for the transmission of impulses which produce a sufficient depth of anaesthesia for surgery.

Acupuncture effects are believed to originate from the prickling of nociceptors in the skin. Since laser beams are supposed to be non-irritant, recent claims by acupuncturists for the efficacy of pulsed He−Ne beams in inhibiting the pathways of pain sensation have added to the controversy and confusion over the whole mechanism of laser-light action.

Kreczi and Klingler (1986) in Austria made a comparison of irradiation of acupoints for 30 seconds by a He−Ne laser and application of a mock laser in 21 patients who were suffering from herniated discs and intervertebral stenosis. The study was repeated after 24 hours when patients who had been lasered received placebo and vice versa. They found that mean pain levels were significantly lower after laser therapy.

Lundeberg et al. (1987) in Stockholm carried out an investigation into whether helium–neon or gallium–arsenide lasers had an analgesic effect and used electro-acupuncture and morphine as controls. Rats were used and the interval before they withdrew their tails after being immersed in hot water was measured. The experiments were repeated after the three treatments were administered. It was found that electro-acupuncture as well as morphine produced a marked increase in response time but neither of the lasers produced any increase.

Synthesis of RNA and DNA
Here again there are claims and counterclaims. In experimental work on the eyes of mice at the Chinese University of Hong Kong, Yew et al. (1982) found that the He–Ne continuous wave laser produced an increase in intercellular substance in the retinas. Their scanning electron microscope also showed an increase in labelled uridine uptake of the pigment epithelium which they considered to be indicative of a possible increase in RNA.

Meyers et al. (1987), in experiments on human lymphocyte cultures, found that radiation by the He–Ne laser exerted no influence on the production of DNA.

Penetration of laser energy
The literature supplied with therapeutic lasers implies that, at their wavelengths, the energy is not absorbed sufficiently by either water or haemoglobin to prevent it from penetrating into the tissues. It then states that He–Ne lasers work at 'superficial skin levels or to a depth of 10 mm' and that 'IR lasers can reach layers as deep as 35 mm or about 3 cm'. An article on the transmission of visible light in tissue can be found in work by Bolin et al. (1984). Their findings suggested that in bovine muscle, at these wavelengths, the distances would be 1.4 mm and 2.8 mm for He–Ne and IR respectively and left the author wondering how the laser could be claimed to influence healing in any subcutaneous tissue.

A study by Lobko et al. (1985) in Moscow raised questions about the hitherto accepted mechanism of the action of laser light. They found that it was not dependent on the light being coherent. Then, Karu (1986) reported equal efficiency of laser and incoherent light in treatment of gastrointestinal lesions. But Boulton and Marshall (1986) in London, after comparing irradiation effects on fibroblast cell lines, reported that the lasered cultures showed a much greater increase in cell numbers than cultures treated with incoherent light.

Karu (1988) proposed that the healing of indolent wounds by laser light is due to its photostimulative effect and that this can initiate cell proliferation in unfavourable conditions such as reduced oxygen concentration, low pH and deficiency in nutrients.

Arrival of new phototherapy machines

Further work at Guy's Hospital by Young et al. (1989) involved a study to ascertain whether light could stimulate the release of mediators of wound repair such as monokines from macrophages. Cells of a macrophage-like cell line were exposed in culture to the following wavelengths of light: 820 nm (coherent and polarized), 660 nm, 870 nm and 880 nm (all non-coherent). After 12 hours the macrophage supernatant was removed and placed on fibroblast cultures. Proliferation was assessed over a 5-day period.

The results showed that wavelengths of 660 nm, 820 nm and 870 nm encouraged the macrophages to release factors that stimulate fibroblast proliferation above the control levels, whereas the 880 nm wavelength either inhibited release of these factors or encouraged release of some inhibitory factors of proliferation.

The evidence that, at certain wavelengths, coherence is not essential was of major practical significance and the report of the phenomenon led to consideration of the use of conventional lamps filtered to the photoactivating wavelength band of about 660 nm. Devices have been developed which provide frequencies from 1 Hz to 1 kHz, with continuous and pulsed modes, and they are being marketed for their analgesic and healing effects in all the common athletic injuries.

Due to the greater divergence of the beam they do not pose the same hazard to the eyesight that is inherent in laser light.

In the commercial world of racing, trainers are contracted to supply runners to tracks and many have various physiotherapy devices, wishfully thinking that they compensate for inadequate exercise and massage and that they are a panacea for every injury. The best that can ensue for the greyhounds is that the device modulates nociceptor activity and produces sufficient analgesia to suppress the clinical manifestations of injury. There is an obligation to try to alleviate pain, but it should always be appreciated that it is a natural response to tissue injury and that its control provides only

symptomatic relief. We also have an obligation to find the cause of
the injury, to remove it and to prevent a recurrence.

Excitement and determination suppress pain

All greyhounds, including those who may be lame on leaving
training kennels, enter a state of sympathetic excitation in antici-
pation of racing on arrival. Behavioural changes from the effects of
adrenaline and noradrenaline release make the detection of slight
lameness difficult or impossible.

All breeds of hounds have an inherent instinct to run and are
observed to take great pleasure from galloping at an early age.
While chasing, the more determined individuals sometimes show
an amazing tolerance to pain. A hound can often be seen falling
over while coursing, get up, and, despite obvious malfunction of a
limb from a fracture or joint dislocation, continue chasing the hare
and sometimes bring it down. On the rare occasions when greyhounds are noticed to be lame at the finish of races on the track,
they are likely to have a major incapacity such as collapse of a hock
joint.

From the time that hounds were first domesticated, our ancestors
received sustenance through their speed for hunting. Even though
we now exploit them for sport and as a betting medium, anyone
concerned for their welfare should remember that we can only give
them the treatment they deserve after assessment of their pain
during a thorough examination, which is not possible while the
animal is on sympathetic drive.

References to Chapter 2

Bassett CAL, Becker RO. (1962) Generation of electric potentials by bone in
    response to mechanical stress. *Science* **137**: 1063–1064
Bassett CAL, Pawluk RJ, Pilla AA. (1974) Augmentation of bone repair by in-
    ductively coupled electromagnetic fields. *Science* **184**: 575–577
Bassett CAL, Pilla AA, Pawluk RJ. (1977) A non-operative salvage of surgically-
    resistant pseudoarthroses and non-unions by pulsing electromagnetic fields. A
    preliminary report. *Clin Orthop* **124**: 128–143
Bassett CAL, Mitchell SN, Schink MM. (1982) Treatment of therapeutically
    resistant non-unions with bone grafts and pulsing electromagnetic fields. *J Bone
    Joint Surg* **64(A)**, 8: 1214–1222
Bassett CAL. (1982) Pulsing Electromagnetic Fields: A new method to modify cell
    behaviour in calcified and noncalcified tissues. *Calcif Tissue Int* **34**: 1–8
Basford JR, Sheffield CG, Mair SD, Ilstrup DM. (1987) Low energy Helium–
    Neon laser treatment of thumb osteoarthritis. *Arch Phys Med Rehab* **68**: 794–
    797

Binder A, Parr G, Hazleman B. *et al.* (1984) Pulsed electromagnetic field therapy of persistent rotator cuff electromagnetic field therapy of persistent rotator cuff tendonitis. *Lancet* 1: 695–698

Bolin FP, Preuss LE, Cain BW. (1984) A comparison of spectral transmittance for several mammalian tissues: effects at PRT frequencies. In: Doiron DR, Gomer CJ (Eds) *Porphyrin Localization and Treatment of Tumours.* Alan R. Liss Inc., New York 211–225

Boulton M, Marshall J. (1986) He–Ne laser stimulation of human fibroblast proliferation and attachment *in vitro. Lasers Life Sci* 1(2): 125–134

Dyson M, Young S. (1986) Effect of laser therapy on wound contraction and cellularity in mice. *Lasers Med Sci* 1: 125–130

England S, Farrell AJ, Coppock JS, Struthers G, Bacon PA. (1989) Low power laser therapy of shoulder tendonitis. *Scand J Rheumatol* 18: 427–431

Frank C, Schachar N, Dittrich D, Shrive N, DeHaas W, Edwards G. (1982) Electromagnetic stimulation of ligament healing in rabbits. *Clin Orthop* 175: 263–271

Gunn HM. (1978) The mean fibre area of the semitendinosus, diaphragm and pectoralis transversus muscles in differing types of horse and dog. *J Anat* 127, (2): 403–414

Gunn HM. (1979) Total fibre numbers in cross sections of the semitendinosus in athletic and non-athletic horses and dogs. *J Anat* 128, (4): 821–828

Gunn HM. (1981) Potential blood supply to muscles in horses and dogs and its relation to athletic ability. *Am J Vet Res* 42, (4): 679–684

Guy PS, Snow DH. (1981) Skeletal muscle fibre composition in the dog and its relationship to athletic ability. *Res Vet Sci* 31: 244–248

Heilmann C, Pette D. (1980) Molecular transformations of sarcoplasmic reticulum in chronically stimulated fast-twitch muscle. In: *Plasticity of Muscle.* Walter de Gruyter, Berlin-New York

Karu TI. (1986) Biological action of low-intensity visible monochromatic light and some of the medical applications. Proceedings of the International Congress on Laser in Medicine and surgery. Bologna, Monduzzi Editore: 25–29

Karu TI. (1988) Molecular Mechanism of the Therapeutic Effect of Low-Intensity Laser Radiation. *Lasers Life Sci* 2(1): 53–74

Kreczi T, Klingler D. (1986) A comparison of laser acupuncture versus placebo in radicular and pseudoradicular pain syndromes as recorded by subjective responses in patients. Acupuncture & Electro-Therapeutics Res., *Int J* 11: 207–216

Lievens P. (1986) The influence of laser-irradiation on the regeneration of venous and lymphatic vessels in the wound healing process. *Lasers Med Surg* Umberto Fornezza (Ed): Cortina International – Verona

Lobko VV, Karu TI, Letokhov VS. (1985) Is low-intensity laser light coherence essential when biological objects are affected.? *Biofizika* 30, (2): 366–371

Lundeberg L, Hode L, Zhou J. (1987) A comparative study of the pain-relieving effect of laser treatment and acupuncture. *Acta Physiol Scand* 131: 161–162

McGillavary GR, Standish WD. (1984) The effects of electrical stimulation on tendon healing. *Orthop Trans* 8: 65

McKibbin LS, Paraschak DM. (1983) A study of the effects of lasering on chronic bowed tendons. *Lasers Surg Med* 3: 55–59

Mester E, Ludany G, Sellyei M, Tota J. (1968) The stimulating effect of low power laser rays on biological systems. *Laser Review* 1: 3

Mester E, Spiry T, Szende B, Tota JG. (1971) Effects of laser rays on wound healing. *Am J Surg* **122**: 532−535

Mester E, Mester A, Toth J. (1983) Biostimulative effect of laser beams. In: Kazuhiko Atsumin (Ed) *New Frontiers in Laser Medicine and Surgery*. Excerpta Medica, Amsterdam-Oxford-Princeton.

Meyers AD, Joyce J, White RA. *et al.* (1987) Biostimulation of wound healing *in vivo* by a He−Ne laser. *Lasers Surg Med* **6**: 540−542

Mulier JC, Spaas F. (1980) Out-patient treatment of surgically resistant non-unions by induced currents. *Arch Orthop Trauma Surg* **97**: 293−297

Pflug JJ. (1975) Intermittent compression in the management of swollen legs. *Practitioner* **215**: 69

Rochkind S, Nissan M, Bar-Nea L, *et al.* (1987) Response of peripheral nerve to He−Ne laser: experimental studies. *Lasers in surgery and medicine* **7**: 441−443

Salmons S, Vrbová G. (1969) The influence of activity on some contractile characteristics of mammalian fast and slow muscle. *J Physiol* **201**: 535−549

Schmallbruch H. The morphology of regeneration of skeletal muscle in the rat. *Tissue Cell* **8**: 673−692

Siebert W, Seichert N, Siebert B, Wirth CJ. (1987) What is the efficacy of 'soft' and 'mid' lasers in therapy of tendinopathies? A double-blind study. *Arch Orthop and Traumatic Surgery* **106**: 358−363

Silver IA, Mccullagh KG, Lanyon LE, Goodship AE, Perry G, Williams IF. (1982) The firing of horses: project **188**: Department of Pathology, University of Bristol

Sturmer KM, Weiss H, Schmit-Neurburg KP. (1985) *Increase of Haversian Remodelling by Electromagnetically Induced Alternating Current*. 5th edn, A.M. Brags, Boston, USA

Summer W, Patrick MK. (1964) *Ultrasonic Therapy*. Elsevier Publishing Company, Amsterdam-London-New York

Walker J. (1983) Relief from chronic pain by low power laser irradiation. *Neurosci Lett* **43**: 339−344

Walker JB, Akhanje LK. (1985) Laser-induced somato-sensory evoked potentials: evidence of photosensitivity in peripheral nerves. *Brain Res* **344**: 281−285

Wu W, Ponnudurai R, Katz J, Pott CB, Chilcoat R, Uncini A, Rapoport S, Wade P, Mauro A. (1987) Failure to confirm report of light-evoked response of peripheral nerve to low power helium−neon laser light stimulus. *Brain Res* **401**: 407−408

Yamada H, Kameya T, Abe N, Miyahara K. (1989) *Low Level Laser Therapy in Horses*. John Wiley & Sons, Chichester 31−35

Yew DT, Ling Wong SL, Chan Yau-wa (1982) Stimulating effect of the low dose laser − A new hypothesis *Acta Anat* **112**: 131−136

Young S, Bolton P, Dyson M, Harvey W, Diamantopoulos C. (1989) Macrophage responsiveness to light therapy. *Lasers Surg Med* **9**: 497−505

3 / Massage and Passive Movement

Massage in the context of this text, refers to 'moving' the soft tissues of the body either with the hands or using suitable machines.

General effects
- Improvement of circulatory flow.
- Reduction of oedema.
- Reduction of muscle spasm.
- Temporary analgesia due to reduction of muscle spasm and reduction of oedema.
- Mobilization of adherent tissue (friction).
- Stretching of contractions (friction).

Massage technique

Hand massage. The hands should mould to the body contour; for small animals, one hand should support as the other works. The hands should be relaxed, the pressure and movement coming from the arm and shoulder. The strokes should be directed to influence venous return (sometimes the lie of the coat may make this impossible).

Massage should be directed over and around areas of muscle spasm. This spasm is located via your 'sense of touch' or as an expression of irritation by the animal when the tissue is palpated. The strokes may be linear, circular or direct compression (Fig. 3.1, Page 26). Massage for 10−30 minutes daily.

Friction massage. The stroke is small and deep and is performed by using the tip of one finger reinforced by a second (Figs 3.2 & 3.3). The movement is across the linear direction of the tissue fibres. The skin and underlying tissue must move as one.

This technique should be followed by general massage to the area. Friction massage should be given on alternate days for 3−7 minutes followed by 15−20 minutes general massage.

Ice massage. Local areas can be massaged with a hand-held ice cube or cube frozen around a 'lolly stick' (see Chapter 4).

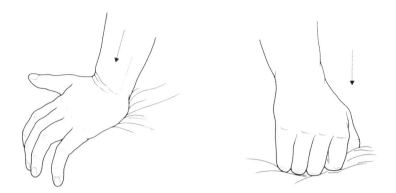

Fig. 3.1 Compression for deep structures. Mould the hands to the underlying structure.

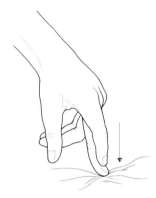

Fig. 3.2 Finger massage to a deep structure.

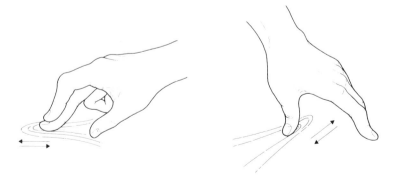

Fig. 3.3 Finger position for friction. Work across the longitudinal direction of underlying fibres.

Machine massage. (Figs 3.4–3.6) The machines have a series of fitments and vibrate rather than massage. The massage machine is probably the only therapeutic device which can safely be used by an 'unqualified' person. As in all cases, a clinical examination should be performed and a diagnosis made prior to treatment.

Technique
- Fit the patient with a muzzle or a bib.
- The machines are mains operated.
- Choose the appropriate fitment.

Allow the animal to become accustomed to both the noise and feel of the machine by using it over an area that is pleasurable (e.g. the neck of the horse). Move the machine in the linear direction of the fibres of the underlying tissue, maintaining a firm even

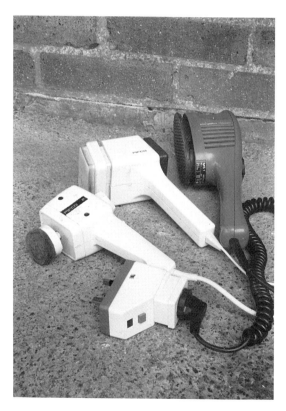

Fig. 3.4 Massage machines. Note the use of a circuit breaker plug.

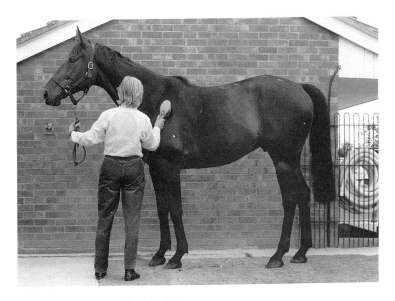

Fig. 3.5 Massage for a shoulder injury.

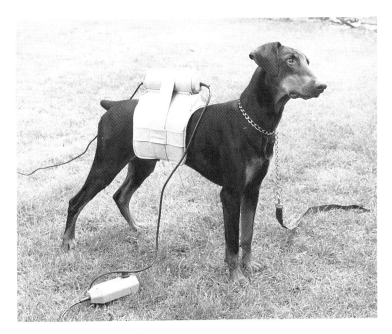

Fig. 3.6 Niagra therapy unit.

pressure. The pressure must be greater over areas of muscle bulk than over bony prominences. Treat for 20–30 minutes daily, twice daily where possible.

INDICATIONS FOR MASSAGE
Oedema in muscle, joints or soft tissue.
Muscle tears.
Muscle sprains, 'pulls'.
Muscle tension/spasm.
Above and below fracture sites, e.g. bulbs of heels for cannon or pastern fractures.

CONTRAINDICATIONS
Infection in an area.
Fracture sites.
Haemarthrosis.
Metastatic disease.

Liniments and rubs
There are a variety of proprietory rubs and liniments available; but there is little evidence to substantiate the claims made by the manufacturers. The massage given at the time of application assists circulatory flow.

Table 3.1 Common liniments and rubs.

Aloe Vera (herbal rub)	Calcium, magnesium, sodium, potassium, copper, iron, manganese, phosphorus, reducer sugars
Arnica (herbal rub)	Arnicia, arnisterin, inolin tennin
Green oils	Parachlorometaxylenol 0/2% w/v Oil of turpentine 28% w/v Arachis oil 30% w/v
Movelat (cream or gel)	Corticosteroids, heparinoid, salicylic acid
Tensolvet	Sodium heparin, 2 hydroxyethyl, salicylate
Trisogel	Sodium heparin, 2 hydroxyethyl, salicylate
Xylocaine ointment	Lignocaine, hydrochloride

All can be rubbed (massaged) over and around the areas of soft tissue damage. They should be used with caution and care; and the user (often the client), finding that one does not work, should not switch to another product without washing the area thoroughly to ensure all traces of the previous product have been removed. Failure to do this may cause a severe local reaction similar, in some instances, to that achieved by the application of the famous 'Irish Red' blister.

Passive movement

Passive movements are a means of retaining and/or regaining joint mobility; they should be performed after the application of heat and massage. The joint is moved by the therapist through as full a range as is possible. There is no muscle action.

It has been shown, by researchers in North America [2] that CPM (continuous passive motion) results in less muscle loss post trauma, due to the stimulation of joint proprioceptors. In cases where damage to the intra-articular cartilage has occurred, regeneration of primitive articular cartilage has been demonstrated following a course of CPM [3].

Technique for passive movement (Figs 3.7−3.9)

The joints above and below the joint to be treated are fixed, where possible. The joint is then moved gently through a full range of

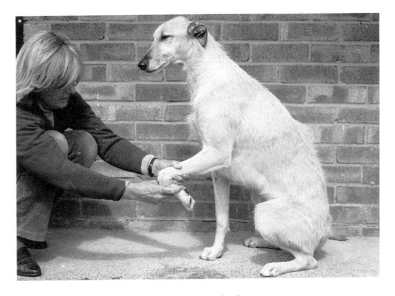

Fig. 3.7 Passive movement. Flexion to a sprained carpus.

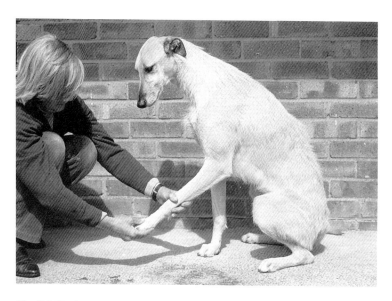

Fig. 3.8 Passive movement. Extension to a sprained carpus.

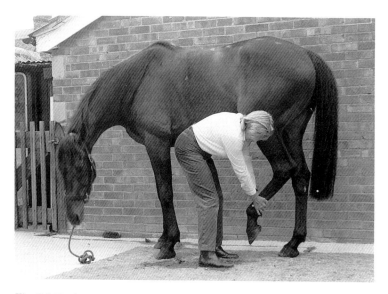

Fig. 3.9 Passive movement to a stiff hock. The stifle joint is fixed against the operator's shoulder to limit the movement of the hock. Note that the operator's hands are *above* the fetlock joint.

movement. If restriction of movement is present, gentle 'over-pressure' is applied at the end of the range.

INDICATIONS
Joint inflammation.
Osteoarthritic joint disease.
Joints with restricted movement following trauma.

CONTRAINDICATIONS
Congenital dislocations of joints.
Fractures involving joints.
Recent haemarthrosis: wait 3−5 days.

4 / Heat and Cold

The external application of heat to the body surface gives rise to changes within tissue. These are either local or general and their extent is governed by the type of heat delivered and the size of the area treated (Fig. 4.1). Artificial sources for the delivery of heat to tissue include hot packs, heated pads, hot water bottles and lamps.

Hot packs and wet heat
Proprietory packs are available, designed to be soaked in boiling water; they retain heat for up to 20 minutes (see Appendix 2).

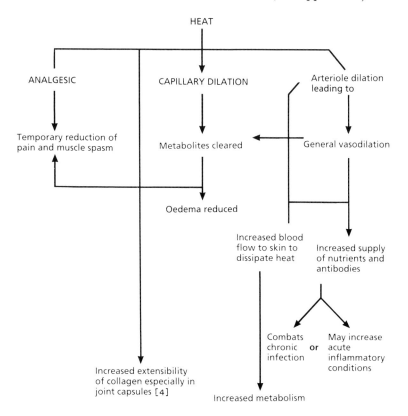

Fig. 4.1 A summary of the application of local external heat after achieving an approximate increase of $39°-44°C$ in the tissue treated.

Hot towels and wet heat

Technique
Place pack or towel in boiling water, squeeze all excess water out of
the pack or towel by placing it in a dry towel and wringing that
towel. Test for comfortable warmth and apply to area of injury. If
appropriate, bandage in place and leave for 20 minutes.

Hot water bottle and dry heat
Small animals will lie comfortably on a hot water bottle placed in
their basket. Cover the bottle with a towel as direct contact can
burn. The animal may be too weak to move.

Electrically heated pads
The pads contain an element which when plugged into an electrical
source emits thermal energy. Some pads run off the mains electricity, others can be preheated.

Rugs
The 'Chaud Cheval' rug is designed with pockets in which infrared
elements are sited. The pads are heated from an external electrical
source (there is a fitment for plugging into a car cigarette lighter).
The rug is available in two sizes: one suitable for a horse, the other
for a greyhound sized dog.

Wraps
Vulkan leg wraps and back packs are manufactured from a material
that acts on a similar principal to the divers' 'dry suit'. Heat is
retained locally by the nature of this material.

Infrared lamps
Infrared generators may be luminous or non-luminous. Non-
luminous units emit 90% long rays with a wavelength of between
15 000 and 770 nm. Approximately 59% of the rays are absorbed in
the superficial epidermis, 6.4% penetrate to the deep part of the
epidermis, the remaining 34% are reflected. Luminous units emit
70% short infrared rays (770–4000 nm wavelength), 4.8% visible
rays, 1% ultraviolet and 24% long infrared rays.
• 34% of the short infrared is reflected.
• 20% is absorbed in the superficial epidermis.

- 16% is absorbed in the deep epidermis.
- 19% reaches the dermis.
- 11% penetrates the subcutaneous tissue.

Luminous infrared lamps are the normal source of heat used in animal clinics. In order to be effective the lamps should be positioned to allow the rays to strike the body surface at an angle of 90°. All lamps should have a wire grill covering the element.

Technique
Position the animal and then the lamp, ensuring that if the animal moves there is no danger of accidental contact with the body surface. Remove any metal that may overheat (collar or harness fittings). There are no set treatment times, but a minimum of 15–20 minutes is suggested unless manufacturers' instructions indicate otherwise.

INDICATIONS
General malaise.
Post trauma.
Following surgery.
Sprains and muscle stiffness.
Colic.

CONTRAINDICATIONS
Impaired sensation. In the author's experience the majority of infrared lamps are sited, particularly in horse establishments, so high above the patient that they are of no practical use.

Sunlight
Due to their living conditions, many animals are denied the ability to absorb natural sunlight. The following artificial sources are available.
Ultraviolet from Ultra Vitalux bulbs or a similar source (see Appendix 2).
Full spectrum lights. Fluorescent tubes producing a spectrum similar to natural sunlight (see Appendix 2).

Cradle solariums containing both infrared and ultraviolet lights are available. The 'hoop' of the cradle ensures a 90° angle to the body surface (Fig. 4.2a,b).

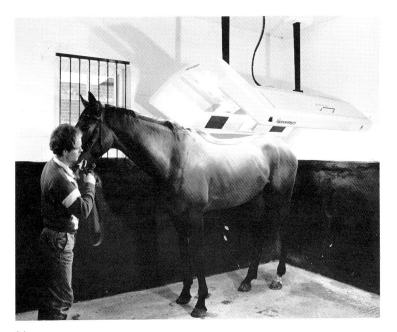

(a)

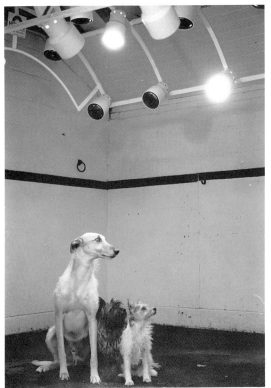

(b)

Fig. 4.2 (a) Hippolarium. (b) Radiant heat and sunlight cradle.

Technique
To ensure maximum absorption, position the lights in such a way that as much surface area as possible is able to receive the light rays at an angle of 90° and a distance of 50−75 cm (approximately 20−30 inches.). Exposure to ultraviolet light should start with 3−5 minutes daily and work up to 15−20 minutes over a 3-week period.

INDICATIONS
Any malaise or injury.

CONTRAINDICATIONS
Light-sensitive conditions. NB: check the manufacturer's instructions before use of therapeutic lights as times vary with the type of element in the bulb.

Cold
The use of cold to control and/or reduce 'filling' particularly in legs is age old, dating back to Hippocrates. Standing a horse in a stream (with a reasonably firm base) is probably the original method of employing cold.

Effects of cold
Immediate vaso-constriction, reducing fluid exudate.
Decrease in tissue temperature. Recent research has shown [5] that the reduction of the oxygen supply to an area, following injury, affects uninjured cells. Cold reduces tissue activity and the oxygen requirement of local undamaged cells decreases; thus, these cells are able to remain competent in a reduced oxygen environment.
Increased circulatory flow in the deep arteries adjacent to the area of damage. As an area becomes unacceptably cold the thermo-regulating mechanism in the cortex is alerted, the deep arterial vessels in the area dilate and arterial blood flow to the area increases.
Known as the 'Hunting Response', this reflex dilation described in 1930 by Lewis *et al.* [6] occurs after 5−10 minutes of cold application, continues for 20−30 minutes and then subsides slowly.

Techniques of cold application for horses
1 *The running stream.* The depth of water determines the height to which the limb can be treated. A pen built in a preferably fast

running stream, enables a horse to be stood in water for varying times and is labour free (Fig. 4.3).

2 *Whirlpool tubs.* Crushed ice can be added. Treats to knee or hock level. The horse is 'persuaded' to place the injured leg into the container. On the first occasion it is better to add the water slowly after the horse has become accustomed to the container.

- Turn on the motor for water activation when the horse has accepted the feel of the water.
- Treat for 20−30 minutes.

3 *Wellie boots.* Crushed ice can be added. Treats to knee/hock level. A less expensive and sophisticated method of creating a similar effect to the Whirlpool tub.

- Persuade the horse to place a leg in each boot.
- Fill with water, adding crushed ice if wished.
- Activate pump.
- Treat for 20−30 minutes.

1, 2 and 3 all combine massage with cold.

4 *Hosing.* Any area can be treated. Run cold water over the injured area for 15−20 minutes from a hose pipe connected to the cold tap.

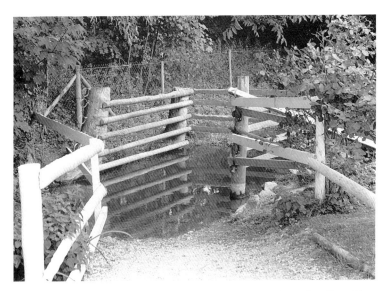

Fig. 4.3 Pen constructed in a running strem. The water depth can be adjusted by a sluice

5 *Cold bandaging* for the horse and dog. This technique can only be used to treat limbs. The bandages are designed in materials that, when damped and placed in the deep freeze, reduce to and remain at a temperature of 6°C after 10 minutes (Fig. 4.4). After removing the bandage from the freezer, the low temperature can be retained by storing in a freezer bag provided for 12 hours.

Apply the bandage to the injured area of the limb or body and leave in place according to the manufacturer's instructions. Each type of bandage varies slightly in formula and melting time.

6 *Frozen gamgee or cotton wool pads* for the horse and dog.

This technique can be used to treat any area. Take a large lump of cotton wool or gamgee, dampen and mould to the limb or

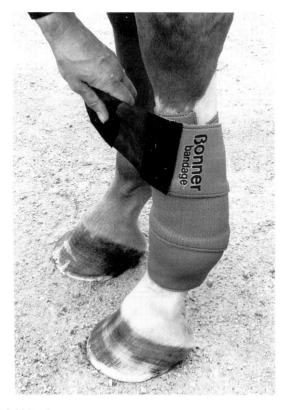

Fig. 4.4 Cold bandage.

injured area. Freeze the shape in the deep freeze. Apply to the injured area over a towel to avoid an ice burn.

7 *Ice massage* for the horse and dog. This technique can be used to treat any area (see Chapter 3). An ice cube, hand-held, or frozen around an 'ice lolly' stick can be employed for a local ice massage.

INDICATIONS FOR COLD APPLICATION
'Fillings' in legs and joints.
Local oedema.
Haematoma formation.

CONTRAINDICATIONS
Open wounds.
Fractures.
Areas where there may be a nerve involvement: sensory or motor.

Contrast bathing
Vaso-constriction on application of cold ⎫ = increased
Vaso-dilation on application of heat   ⎭   circulatory flow

Technique
Soak a towel or cloth in iced water, wring dry and apply for 3 minutes. Soak a towel in boiling water, wring dry and apply for 3 minutes. Repeat cold and heat alternately for 20–30 minutes to area of damage.

INDICATIONS
Soft tissue damage.
Haematoma.
'Filled' joints.
'Filled' legs.

CONTRAINDICATIONS
Open wounds.
Infections.

5 / Magnetic Field Therapy

In the 1960s research at the University of Saarbrucken described the effects of a pulsed magnetic field (PMF) on tissue [7]. The effects of magnetic forces on man using magnetite or lodestone were used in the Middle Ages.

Today electromagnetism is created by passing a current through a coil circling a suitable conducting material; the measurement unit of intensity in PMF is the Tesla (T). The calibration of intensity is calculated as a percentage of 1 T in most therapeutic apparatus, 100% being equivalent to 10 MT or 100 gauss (G). A pulsed magnetic field is achieved by programming the control unit to emit current bursts, referred to as pulses.

The number of pulses per second or frequency is the most important parameter in PMF, the choice of frequency determining the biological effects. This parameter is measured in hertz (Hz): 1 Hz denotes a frequency of 1 pulse per second. Therapeutic purposes require a delivery from 1 to 50 Hz.

Effects

Cellular effects. The complexity of the cell is not yet clearly understood but it has been demonstrated that the surface potential of cells alter from the accepted 'normal' when a tissue is diseased or injured. It appears that by passing a PMF through tissue, provided that the intensity and pulse frequency selected are 'in tune' with the cells whose surface potential is temporarily incorrect, the alternating field may help to re-establish the correct surface potential of the cells, and thus restore normal function.

Increased vascularity. Measurement has shown increased vascularity and a rise in the partial pressure of oxygen in tissue [7] treated with PMF. Healing is assisted by the improved circulatory flow and an increase in the partial pressure of oxygen. Acceleration of the removal of metabolic waste products is also achieved.

Pain relief. Melzack and Wall (1965) [8] were the first to demonstrate that by subjecting large nerve fibres to selected wave forms, pain perception can be significantly reduced. Some of the PMF frequencies achieve this situation.

Static fields and battery-operated magnetic fields

Magnetic pads
These pads are suitable for large or small animals and they can be strapped or bandaged into place. The material contains a series of magnets arranged in a manner designed to create a perpetual magnetic field of around 680 gauss (G). The ceramic coating gives flexibility allowing the pad to mould over uneven surfaces. The penetrable depth is approximately 17 mm.

Blue boot
Battery operated. Designed in USA specifically for the treatment of sore shins; the designers claim the field produced is specific for bone healing. Their results show early callus formation (X-ray and bone density proof). The Blue boot was **not** designed for soft tissue repair. Soft tissue cells are influenced by frequencies that differ from those that influence bone cells [9].

Mains-operated units
The Magneto Pulse and System MFT are the two units currently available in the UK.

The generator delivers current to four magnets which can be attached to appropriately sized rugs for treatment of the animal's body, or singly can be wrapped around a limb or adapted to create an all-embracing magnetic field (Fig. 5.1).

The reduction in pain following MFT does not mean the tissue has returned to pre-injury state. The analgesic effect will give an illusion of recovery, therefore resume work with caution.

Technique
Magnetic pads (all animals)
• Clean skin area thoroughly. If a 'rub' or 'wash' has been used; blistering will occur if there is an agent between the skin and pad.
• Bandage or strap pad over injured area. (Small dogs will lie on pads if placed in their basket.)
• Leave *in situ* for up to 12 hours.
• Remove pad and inspect skin.

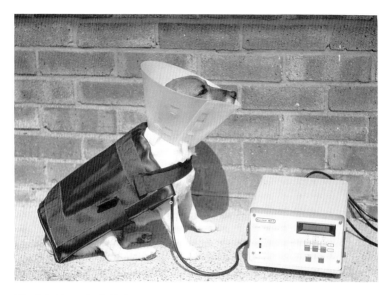

Fig. 5.1 Magnetic field therapy. Terrier with acute back pain.

- Replace pad.
- Use until condition improves (4−10 days).

Blue boot (large animals)

- Charge unit overnight.
- Strap in place over area of shin soreness.
- Leave for 2 hours.
- Repeat daily until healing occurs (10−15 days).

Magneto pulse or System MFT (all animals) (Fig. 5.2)

- Use a bib or a muzzle.
- Check for and remove any metal from the path of the MFT
- Position animal so that it cannot move.
- Place magnets (or magnet) in desired positions.
- Attach leads to cable drums.
- Position unit safely.
- Attach to mains.
- Attach cable drum leads to unit.
- Select time, intensity (G) and frequency (Hz) suitable to the condition.
- Switch on.
- Treat once daily. Time to manufacturer's instructions.

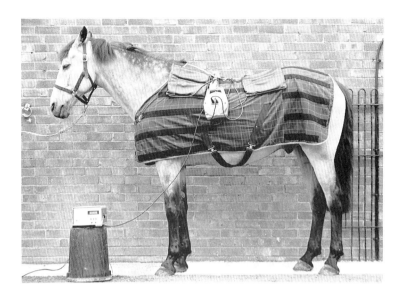

Fig. 5.2 Magnetic field therapy; the magnets are arranged in pairs across the horse's back.

INDICATIONS
Pain relief.
Fractures (is effective through plaster).
Arthritic joints.
Muscle tendon and ligament tears.
Bruising.
NB: Cats, in general, will not tolerate exposure to MFT; the reason has not been established.

CONTRAINDICATIONS (as advised by the manufacturers)
Sepsis.
Acute viral or other infections.
Pregnancy.
NB: All electronic equipment is highly sensitive to magnetic activity.
Do not use within 2 metres of electronic apparatus.

Dosage and times
4–6 Hz reduces oedema.

10 Hz + improves circulatory flow.

25 Hz + affects bone.

See instruction manual for settings appropriate to both condition and control unit. Times vary for each unit.

6 / Muscle Stimulators

Muscle weakness occurs for a variety of reasons.

1 Direct trauma resulting in haematoma formation, loss of elasticity, adhesions or scarring.

2 Sprains or tears in the belly of the muscle, at the origin or insertion, at the musculo-tendinous junction or in the tendon.

3 Disuse atrophy. The reason for disuse atrophy is little understood. Recent work in North America [10] suggests reduction in normal joint function leads to a loss of communication between the joint proprioceptors and the muscles supporting those joints. (It has long been recognized that a strain of the lateral ligament of the human ankle, damaging the proprioceptors located in the lateral ligament, leads to atrophy of the peroneal muscles. Unless exercises, specific for peronei [11], are performed, chronic ankle weakness occurs.)

4 Motor neurone disease.

5 Neuropraxia (Fig. 6.1).

6 Section of motor nerve.

Contrary to general belief, weak muscles do not regain their pre-injury strength unless they are stimulated and exercises specific to the injured muscle or muscle groups are given.

There may be an illusion of recovery as other supporting groups take over the work of the injured muscle often in an imperceptible manner. However, the change of function creates secondary problems: joint strain, ligament strain and back problems.

Koch (USSR) [12] has shown that weak or recovering motor units can only 'fire' 10 times, the unit then being unable to fire correctly without a rest period of 1 minute to allow the muscle to 're-fuel' or recover.

Until recently the faradic-type current was the only available method of stimulating muscle. The method is out-dated. Good results can only be achieved if the active electrode is placed directly over the motor point of the muscle (generally sited in the middle of the longitudinal axis of the muscle) and, due to the 'pricking' sensation created under the electrodes, it is difficult to persuade the animal to tolerate a current flow of sufficient strength to stimulate deep muscles. The isolation of a single muscle requires a very

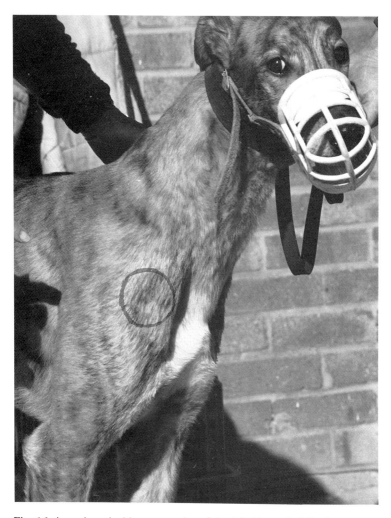

Fig. 6.1 A greyhound with gross wasting of the deltoid muscle following a neuropraxia.

precise anatomical knowledge. Faradism requires that the motor nerve be intact.

Diagnostic faradism

Stimulation of damaged muscle causes pain, the animal flinching or trying to move. The electrode used is moved slowly over the muscle group in an attempt to isolate the area of damage by the

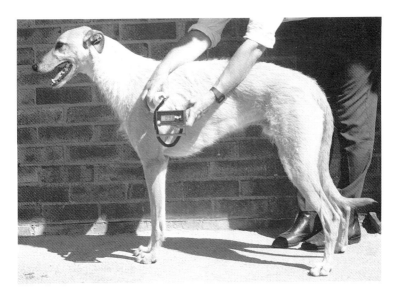

Fig. 6.2 Measuring the deltoid muscle with a myometer.

reaction of the patient. This method has been surplanted by the use
of the EMG and the myometer (Fig. 6.2).

Trophic electrical stimulation
Neurophysiological research has enabled efficient new muscle
stimulators to be designed. These new machines deliver a signal
which mimics the firing patterns and frequency of the motor
neurone. The injured muscle regains the pre-injury density in the
capillary bed, is able to utilize oxygen and to recover the pre-injury
state. De-nervated muscles will respond to this type of stimulation
if the motor end plate is intact.

   An analysis of healthy motor neurones has revealed the following
pulse/second requirement.

5–15 pulses/second   Improvement of muscle tone, aids joint
                      mobility and support.
                      Improvement of capillary bed density leading
                      to [13] improved fatigue resistance. (The
                      natural firing frequency received by slow
                      glycolytic oxidative muscle fibres is 10 pulses/
                      second.)

15−25 pulses/second Assists in promoting endurance [14]. (The
                     natural firing frequency received by the fast
                     oxidative glycolytic muscle fibres.)
30−40 pulses/second Utilized to strengthen muscle.

The stimulators employ a waveform that embraces the required
pulse/second requirements.

Techniques
Test every machine on yourself before treating an animal. Place the
electrodes over a muscle group, switch on machine and increase
intensity until a contraction occurs.

Preparation for animal treatment
The current will not generally penetrate a thick or waterproof coat.
Work the transmitting gel well into the coat before applying the
electrodes; failure to achieve contraction may require the coat to be
clipped. The density of a greyhound's coat is the maximum that
will allow the even passage of the current.

Faradism
The amount of skin sensation created by the passage of this current
is not well tolerated by some animals.

Faradic stimulation (suitable for large or small animal treatment).
The unit houses the circuit. Control knobs regulate the number of
contractions per minute and intensity of stimulus. Two pads, a
large 'indifferent' pad and a similar 'active' pad are attached by
leads to the unit. (Battery operated machines are available.)

Method for faradism
Position the animal.
Position the unit.
Decide the placement of the large indifferent pad, the area just behind
    the shoulders is usual.
Soak the animal's coat in the area chosen for the indifferent pad.
Soak the pad in weak saline; it is the best conductor and reduces the
    skin sensation.
Strap firmly into place with the 'girth' provided.
Soak the coat over the area to be treated.

Soak the active pad, also in weak saline.

Hold the active pad firmly over the motor point of the muscle to be treated.

Turn up the intensity slowly until a contraction occurs.

Allow 10 contractions, turn intensity down and move the active pad to another motor point.

Treat for 20–30 minutes daily. Two 15-minute sessions are preferable to one long session.

The greater the intensity of the current, the stronger the muscle contraction. Vary the length of time the muscle remains contracted from a long slow hold to a short quick twitch.

The Transeva (not suitable for small animals)

The late Sir Charles Strong designed a machine based on the faradic principle, the wave form changed to reduce skin sensation. The method of application is similar to faradism but is not specific to one muscle. The weak or injured area is lubricated with gel and the active pad moved continuously, in a circular motion, over a group of muscles.

The Animate (large or small animals)

This is a battery operated unit, similar to but smaller than the Transeva. A pair of similar sized electrode pads supply the current. Gel and position the pads one at either end of the muscle to be treated and keep in place with a firm hand pressure. Switch on the unit and increase intensity to achieve a muscle contraction.

The Orthotron (large or small animals)

This is a small unit powered by a re-chargeable battery with two sets of self-adhering electrodes. Minimal skin sensation occurs even at maximum output. One set of pads or both can be used as required.

Method for Orthotron

Position the animal.

Use a bib or a muzzle.

Place a suitable surcingle around the girth area (the surcingle should have a fitment suitable for the attachment of the unit).

Gel the electrode placement areas.

Position electrodes.

Plug leads into unit.

Turn on machine.

Increase intensity to one pair of electrodes until a suitable contraction occurs.

Increase intensity to the second pair of electrodes when the animal
has settled.

Strap the unit to the surcingle on horse. Ensure that the leads do
not irritate the animal causing skin twitches which could dislodge
the pads.

A horse may be left for the treatment period with a haynet.

Dogs are best with a handler.

A 'bleep' will sound should a pad detach.

Treatment times: 20–30 minutes daily or twice daily for 15
minutes.

DMI mark II and Neurotech NT 2EF (large or small animals)
(Figs 6.3 and 6.4)

These units and all other similar machines are the newest and most
efficient battery operated muscle stimulators. A muscle 'ripple'
occurs rather than a full contraction. The relaxation cycle is slightly
longer than the stimulation cycle, allowing dispersal of any reactive
hyperaemia.

There is minimal skin sensation allowing maximum contraction.
Each unit is fitted with two pairs of electrodes and two intensity
controls. Both pairs of electrodes may be used to stimulate agonist
and antagonist muscles respectively, or two groups can be stimulated
at the same time. A single pair of electrodes may be used effectively
on one muscle only.

Method of DMI mark II and Neurotech NT 2EF

Position the patient.

Check controls are at zero.

Decide the electrode placement.

Gel the areas.

Place one electrode (the negative or active) over or near the motor
point of the muscle.

Place the second electrode (passive or positive) over the muscle
bulk or distal to the first.

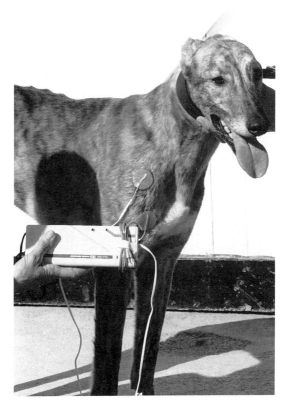

Fig. 6.3 Muscle stimulation to the deltoid muscle, using the Neurotech 2 EF machine.

Position the second set of electrodes if required.
Increase the intensity of one pair of electrodes until a suitable contraction is achieved.
Repeat with the second pair of electrodes.

Attach the unit to a suitable surcingle on the horse. Horses may be left if checked regularly but dogs should not be unattended. Treat for up to 30 minutes. The stimulus is soothing and most animals appear to relax and tolerate the treatment well. Active exercise will complement muscle stimulation. The nature of the case will determine at what stage active exercise should be included in the treatment regime; as a general rule it can be assumed that the earlier the better.

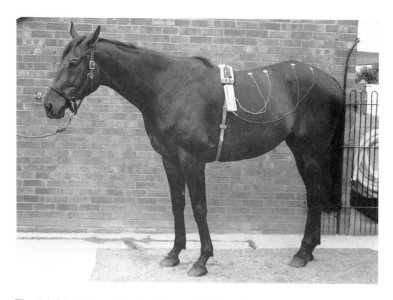

Fig. 6.4 Stimulation using the Neurotech 2EF unit to the longissimus muscle and the middle gluteal muscles.

INDICATIONS FOR MUSCLE STIMULATION

Fractures: stimulate supporting muscle groups.

Tendon injury: stimulate parent muscle.

Joint strain: stimulate supporting muscle groups.

Sacro-iliac joint subluxation: stimulate supporting muscle groups.

Muscle tears: stimulate to avoid adhesions and maintain tone.

Nerve section or neuropraxia: stimulate affected muscles to maintain tone.

Haematoma: stimulate muscles involved to disperse haematoma and avoid adhesions.

Post surgery: stimulate groups weak from disuse atrophy.

Road traffic accident: stimulate muscle groups involved to regain full limb function.

CONTRAINDICATIONS

Infection.

Neoplasia.

Motor neurone disease.

Transcutaneous electrical nerve stimulators (TENS) (Fig. 6.5)
Transcutaneous electrical nerve stimulators (TENS) or Doctor
Pulse are both used as pain suppressors and are similar units with
differing trade names. The small battery operated units supplied
with two or four electrodes are designed to deliver a current con-
sisting of a series of pulses. The number of pulses per second
(pps) and intensity can both be adjusted to block pain perception.

Pain
• Unmyelinated 'C' fibres monitor and record dull, chronic aching
type pain.
• TENS units 'block' 'C' fibre pain.
• Small myelinated 'A' delta fibres monitor and record sharp
red hot, electric type pain. TENS units 'block' 'A' delta fibre pain.

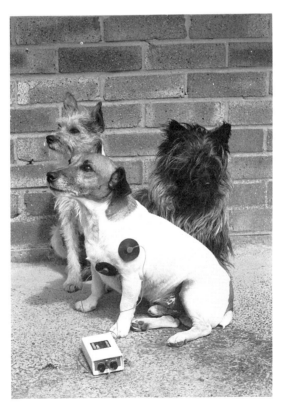

Fig. 6.5 Transcutaneous nerve stimulation to a dog's shoulder.

The gate control theory of Melzac and Wall (1965) [15] is still the most generally accepted hypothesis on pain control; the TENS units have been developed based on this hypothesis. Their theory postulates a neural mechanism located in the dorsal horn of the spinal cord. The somatosensory input is 'blocked' by this mechanism before perception occurs. In order that the TENS units are effective, the source of the pain must be determined. The electrodes are placed so that the current flow passes through the pain source. By adjustment of the pps it is possible to achieve an analgesic effect.

Technique
Determine the source of pain.
Position the animal.
Gel the electrodes.
Position to allow current to flow through the source of pain.
Turn on.
Increase intensity until a small muscle 'flick' occurs.
Turn down to just below the muscle flick.
Adjust pulses/second according to manufacturer's instructions.
Treat according to the manufacturer's instructions.

INDICATIONS
Chronic pain as in arthritic conditions.

CONTRAINDICATIONS
Sepsis or any infection.

TENS may be used to control pain in metastatic disease.

Motor points for common muscle injuries in the horse

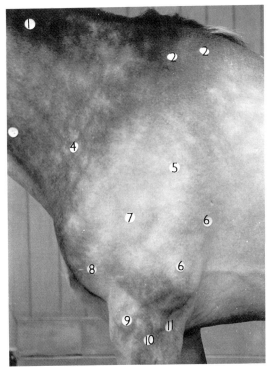

Fig. 6.6 Left lateral view, shoulder area.

1 *Rhomboideus*: stimulate after neck or wither problems.

2 *Trapezius*: stimulate after shoulder problems.

4 *Infraspinatus*: stimulate after neck, shoulder and leg problems.

5 *Supraspinatus*: stimulate after neck, shoulder and leg problems.

6 *Long and lateral head triceps*: stimulate after shoulder and leg problems, also after radial palsy.

7 *Deltoideus*: stimulate after shoulder and leg problems, also following radial palsy.

8 *Cleidobrachialis*: stimulate after shoulder problems.

9 *Extensor carpi radialis*: stimulate after knee and tendon problems.

10 *Extensor digitorium communis*: stimulate after knee and tendon problems.

11 *Extensor carpi ulnaris*: stimulate after shoulder and tendon problems.

Motor points for common muscle injuries in the horse

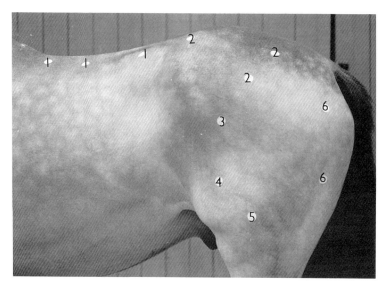

Fig. 6.7 Left lateral view, back and quarters.

1 *Longissimus*: stimulate after all back and pelvic problems.
2 *Gluteus medius*: stimulate after all back, pelvic and hip problems.
3 *Rectus femoris*: stimulate after hip, hock and stifle problems.
4 *Vastus lateralis*: stimulate after hip, hock and stifle problems.
5 *Gastrocnemius*: stimulate after hip and hock problems.
6 *Semitendinosus*: stimulate after a tear in the muscle (fibrotic myopathy), also after hip or hock problems.

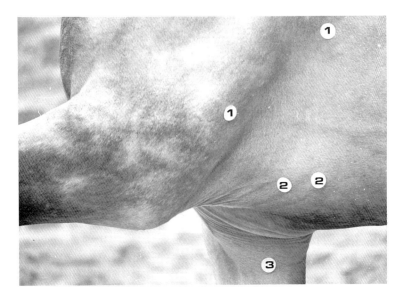

Fig. 6.8 Left pectoral area.

1 *Triceps*: stimulate after shoulder and leg problems.
2 *Deep pectoral*: stimulate after shoulder, elbow or leg problems.
3 *Flexor carpi ulnaris*: stimulate after shoulder, elbow or leg problems.

Motor points for common muscle injuries in the horse

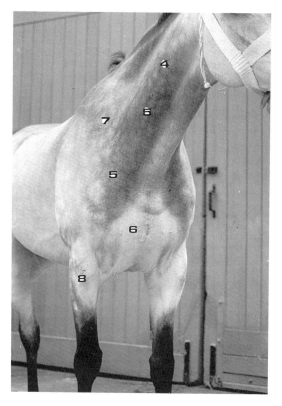

Fig. 6.9 Right rostal view.

4 *Sternocephalic*: stimulate after shoulder or neck problems.
5 *Brachiocephalic*: stimulate after neck or shoulder problems.
6 *Superficial pectoral*: stimulate after any shoulder problems.
(Weakness of this muscle reduces the stability of the foreleg of that side.)
7 *Supraspinatus*: stimulate after shoulder or neck problems.
8 *Extensor carpi radialis*: stimulate after shoulder problems or radial palsy.

Motor points for common muscle injuries in the horse

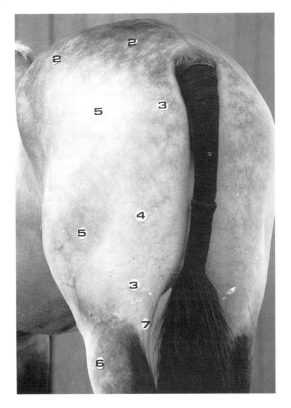

Fig. 6.10 Left caudolateral view.

2 *Gluteus medius*: stimulate after lumbar spine or pelvic problems.
3 *Semitendinosus*: stimulate after hip or hock problems.
4 *Semimembranosus*: stimulate after hip or hock problems.
5 *Biceps femoris*: stimulate after hip or hock problems. (A tear in 3, 4 and/or 5 is a common injury, fibrosis or calcification of the tear is common. Ultrasound in conjunction with muscle stimulation is beneficial.)
6 *Extensor digitorum lateralis*: stimulate after stifle problems.
7 *Gastrocnemius*: stimulate after hip or hock problems, also if a curb is causing problems.

Motor points for common injuries in the dog

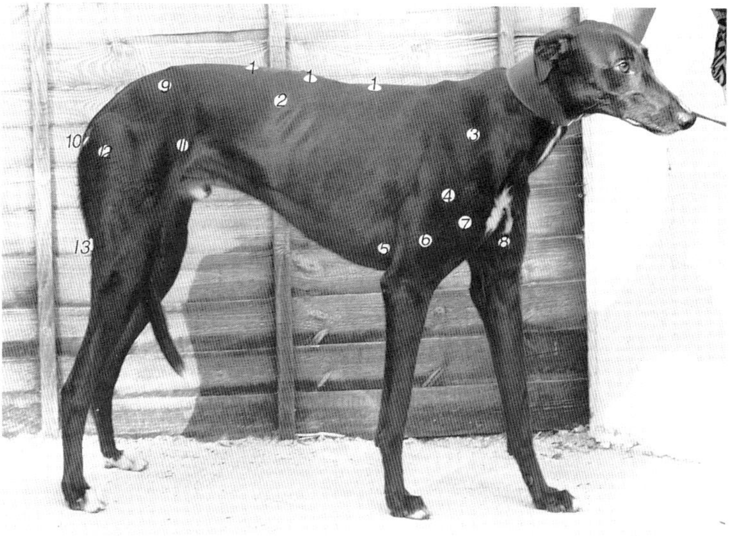

Fig. 6.11 Right lateral view.

1 *Longissimus dorsi*: stimulate after all back problems; if the weakness is bilateral stimulate both sides simultaneously.

2 *Psoas*: stimulate after all back and/or pelvic problems.

3 *Trapezius*: stimulate after all shoulder problems.

4 *Deltoideus:* stimulate after all shoulder and elbow problems.

5 *Superficial pectoral*: stimulate after all shoulder and forelimb problems. (Weakness results in instability of the limb.)

6 *Triceps*: stimulate after all shoulder and elbow problems.

7 *Brachiocephalicus* (cleidobrachialis): stimulate after all shoulder and/or elbow problems.

8 *Brachiocephalicus* (cleidobrachialis): stimulate after all shoulder and/or elbow problems.

9 *Gluteus medius*: stimulate after all back, pelvic or hip problems.

10 *Semimembranosus*: stimulate after all hip and/or hock problems.

11 *Sartorius* (whip muscle): stimulate after all back, pelvic or hip problems.

12 *Gluteus superficialis*: stimulate after all back, pelvic or hip problems.

13 *Gracilis*: stimulate after all hip or hock problems. (Weakness results in an unstable pelvic limb.)

Motor points for common injuries in the dog

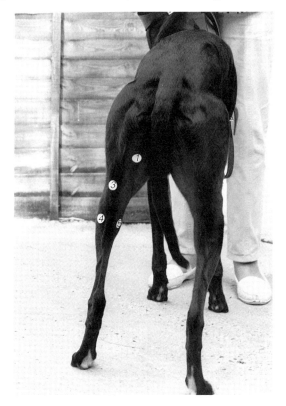

Fig. 6.12 Caudal view.

1 *Gracilis*: stimulate after all hip or hock problems.
3 *Semitendinosus*: stimulate after all hip and hock problems.
4 *Flexor digitorum profundus*: stimulate after all hip and/or hock problems.
5 *Gracilis*: stimulate after all pelvic, hip and/or hock problems.

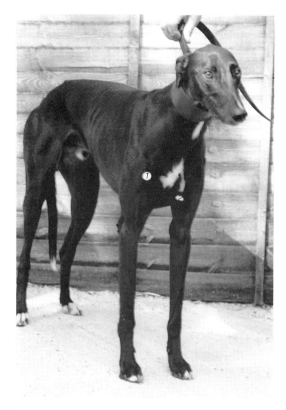

Fig. 6.13 Rostal view.

1 *Supraspinatus*: stimulate after all shoulder and forelimb lameness.
2 *Superficial pectoral*: stimulate after all shoulder and forelimb problems.

7 / Therapeutic Ultrasound

Ultrasound is produced by subjecting a quartz or other type of suitable crystal to bombardment by a high frequency current. The longitudinal compression waves that result have a frequency above that recognized by the human ear. It is important to note that some animals are able to hear higher frequencies than humans (20 kHz is the upper human limit). Distress demonstrated by an animal during treatment could be the result of an ability to register a previously unknown, and therefore unclassified, sound or it may be the result of pain due to an incorrect setting. Check by reducing the W/cm^2.

Ultrasound machines are designed to be powered by either mains electricity or from a rechargeable battery (Figs 7.1 and 7.2). For

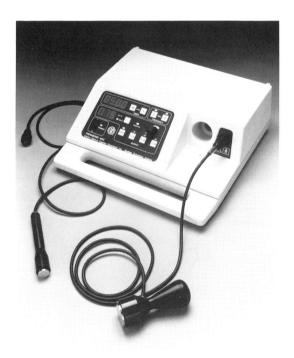

Fig. 7.1 Battery powered ultrasound unit by EMS. Note the two transducers.

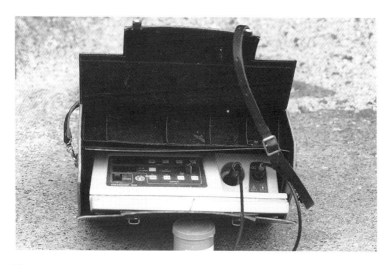

Fig. 7.2 Portable ultrasound in a carrying case. The case hangs on the operators shoulder.

animal treatment the battery operated machine is the obvious choice. A generator produces a high frequency current which is conveyed to the head of the applicator, transducer, by a coaxial cable. The crystal, housed in the transducer head, vibrates in response to the current and sound waves are created. The majority of modern machines can be programmed to operate at either 1 MHz or 3 MHz.

Choice of wavelength
The longitudinal waves of ultrasound cause the cells in their path to oscillate to and fro in the direction of the waves. The wavelength is the distance from the middle of one compression to the middle of the next. At 1 MHz setting, the calculated distance of effective penetration into the tissue is 4 cm. As the frequency rises the effective penetration decreases and at 3 MHz setting, the calculated penetrative depth is 2.5 cm. For superficial lesions a setting of 3 MHz should be selected, but for deep lesions a setting of 1 MHz or 0.75 MHz is required.

Intensity
The intensity of output is measured in watts per square centimetre (W/cm^2). This energy when transmitted to the tissues determines

the rate of oscillation of cells in the path of the beam; dependent on the tissue type to be treated and the effects required, so the W/cm^2 *must* be selected.

Each tissue type offers a differing resistance to the passage of the ultrasonic wave, described as acoustic impedance. The different resistances present at the tissue interfaces cause a rise in thermal energy; this must be taken into account when calculating the W/cm^2. Increasing the W/cm^2 does not increase the depth of penetration; it merely increases the cell agitation and thermal energy.

Pulsed ultrasound
The thermal effects of ultrasound are reduced if a pulsed beam is used. The settings on machines are usually 1:5 or 1:4; some equipment provides a 1:1 ratio. At 1:5 the dosage is 'on' or delivered for one-fifth of the exposure time. Using 1:5 pulsed for 10 minutes means that the patient has received only 2 minutes of actual treatment. The pulsed settings should be selected when treatment is to be given over areas of superficial bone as pulsed settings minimize the thermal effects created at the bony interface.

Effects of ultrasound
Laboratory work [16] has established that ultrasound energy is absorbed at the molecular level. It is the proteins among the molecular constituents of soft tissue that are the major absorbers.
• Nerve protein is sensitive to ultrasound.
• Blood haemoglobin absorbs ultrasound.
• Muscle protein absorbs ultrasound.
• Cell membrane absorbs ultrasound.
As the absorption of energy causes changes in tissue, it is essential to appreciate several points in order to achieve a safe and effective treatment.
• The nature of the condition.
• The tissue type.
• The depth at which the tissue lies.
• The types of tissue between the surface and damaged area.
• The linear direction of the fibres.
• The nature of the surrounding tissue.

Thermal effects. The friction caused by cell movement creates heat.

Providing there is an adequate blood supply, this heat is readily dissipated and will not cause a deep tissue burn.

Extreme caution must be exercised in cases where the blood supply is impaired and/or there is damage to the local nerve supply.

Chemical effects. Nothing significant has been proved in this field.

Electrical effects. Disturbance of the thin layer of ions sited at the boundary between a solid and an electrolytic solution occurs as a result of the 'pressure' of the beam [17].

Effects on bone. Seventy per cent of the energy delivered to bone is reflected to the periosteum. The angle of the reflected energy waves bouncing back off the bone differs from the angle of the arriving energy. The shear stress waves created increase the local heat and, since the periosteum is avascular, no cooling occurs and the excessive heat will cause severe pain. *Treat bony areas with low dosage levels to avoid the danger of pathological fractures.*

Effects on nerve tissue. Studies have shown [18] that specific intensities of ultrasound alter peripheral nerve propagation.

3 W/cm^2 = increase in nerve conduction velocity.
$1-2 \text{ W/cm}^2$ = decrease in nerve conduction velocity.
0.5 W/cm^2 = increase in motor nerve velocity.

Andersen and Herrick have established [18] that 'A' fibres are the least sensitive, 'B' are the most sensitive, with 'C' between 'A' and 'B'.

Phonophoresis
A substance dissolved or suspended in a coupling medium can be driven through the skin into the underlying tissue for depths of up to 50 mm. The use of a continuous beam at 2 W/cm^2 increases the permeability of the cell membrane by 200% and allows for absorption of the substance. Hydrocortisone cream is commonly used as it is useful for treatment of subcutaneous inflammation.

Techniques for testing machines (Fig. 7.3)
The unit can be tested by either:
covering the head of the transducer with gel, or

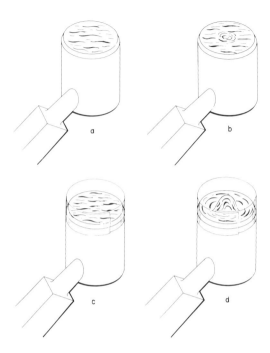

Fig. 7.3 Testing the ultrasound transducer. (a) Cover treatment surface with coupling medium. (b) Turn on the machine, increase the intensity and look for bubbles in the centre of the coupling medium. (c) Make a lip by winding the masking tape around the treatment head and fill with water. (d) Turn on the machine, increase the intensity and the water should cone.

wrapping some masking tape around the head of the transducer
    to form a lip; and filling the so-formed cup with water.
    Turn on the unit and increase the wattage. If the machine is
working the gel will be seen to 'bubble' over the central area of the
transducer surface or the water will be forced into a cone centrally.
    Turn off the unit and wipe off the gel, or tip the water away and
remove the tape.

Animal treatment techniques (Figs 7.4 and 7.5)
Place the animal in a position where it is secure and you can work
    safely before preparing the area to be treated by clipping.
Gel the area thoroughly.
Place the unit in a secure position.
Select pulsed or continous setting.

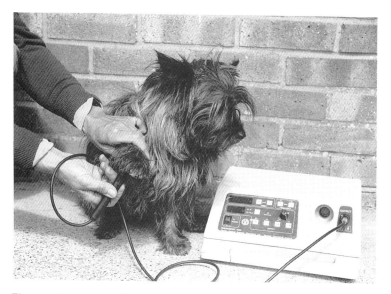

Fig. 7.4 Ultrasound applied to a ligament injury.

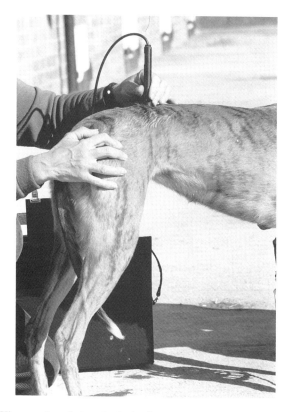

Fig. 7.5 Ultrasound applied to the back of a greyhound following a back injury.

Select the correct Hertz setting (1 MHz or 3 MHz).

Switch on mains supply for mains machine.

Place the correctly sized transducer head over the area to be treated
at a 90° angle to the surface.

Switch on.

Switch on the automatic timer.

Turn up the wattage setting to that appropriate for the condition.

Move the transducer head slowly over the gelled area throughout
the treatment, in either a circular or linear direction.

At the conclusion of the treatment, switch off the machine and
remove to a safe place. Finally wash off and dry the treated area.

Underwater method

It is sometimes considered easier to treat a limb underwater due to
an uneven surface area. Water does not reflect or refract the
ultrasonic beam unless air bubbles are present. Degassed water is
recommended. This method was popular before the introduction of
the small transducer head.

Clip the area of the limb requiring treatment and soak the limb.

Fill a suitable container with water, making certain that there are
no air bubbles.

Place the limb in the container (the jacuzzi tub is suitable).

Rub the area to be treated when it is in the water to ensure no air
is trapped at the base of the hairs.

Put the transducer head in the water.

Direct the beam at right angles to the area to be treated holding the
transducer head 1 cm away from the surface of the limb and
proceed as for the gel method.

Dry with towels at the conclusion of treatment.

INDICATIONS FOR THERAPEUTIC ULTRASOUND
(See pp. 94−108 for treatment times.)

Adhesions between adjacent uninjured tissues occur following
trauma but are reversible.

Joint contractures following trauma.

Loss of elasticity in a joint capsule (there will be improvement in
synovial fluid production) [19].

Tears or damage to ligaments.

Tears or damage to tendons.

Osteoarthritic joints.

Adhesions following metal implants. As ultrasound waves are acoustic not electromagnetic their use in the presence of metal implants is not contraindicated.

Bursitis.

Synovitis.

Sinusitis.

Haematoma. Low doses around the periphery for 48 hours combined with ice and if possible compression prevents organization of exudate. After 48 hours the whole area may be treated with a low dosage to assist reabsorption of the exudate.

Pain and muscle spasm. Ultrasound at intensities of $1-2$ W/cm^2, reduces the nerve conduction of the pain-carrying 'C' fibres. This will reduce muscle spasm and allow the resumption of circulation.

Calcification (calcified myositis) [20]. The excitation of calcium bound to proteins promotes the fragmentation and resorption of calcified masses within soft tissue (an anti-inflammatory injection prior to treatment is of great assistance).

Wound healing. In the absence of bacteria low doses promote the formation of granulation tissue. Ultrasound has been superceded by cold laser therapy in this field.

Fractures. There have been conflicting reports on the effects of ultrasound; it appears that high doses may interfere with the formation of callus. The work of Dyson and Pond suggests low doses do not retard callus formation [16].

Bone. Doses of high intensity ultrasound and over-treatment have resulted in pathological fractures and subperiosteal damage. It is considered that ultrasound given to epiphyseal plates is destructive. It should not be used in cases of epiphysitis.

CONTRAINDICATIONS

Tumours.

Acute infection or sepsis.

Avoid the brain, eyes and reproductive organs.

Heart disease or atherosclerotic conditions.

Tuberculosis of lung or bone.

Epiphysitis.

Fractures.

Coupling media

A medium with a high sound transmissivity is required. Aquasonic or Soni-gel can transmit almost 90% but lanolin-based creams are opaque to ultrasound and cause heating of the transducer head with little or no transmission to tissue occurring.

Dosage

There are no set dosage criteria. The condition must be reviewed daily and experience is the best guide. Treatment can be given once daily for up to 10 days, but it should not exceed two 10-day courses without a 3-week rest. There is no progression of dosage. The dose suitable for the condition is chosen and provided there is no evidence of pain that dosage is adhered to. A rough guideline based on continuous ultrasound is set out below; for pulsed ultrasound calculate according to setting.

Pain relief.
   $1.0-1.5$ W/cm^2 to nerve fibres for $3-5$ minutes (3 MHz).
   $0.5-1$ W/cm^2 continuous to nerve roots and ganglia for $3-4$ minutes (3 MHz).
Reducing adhesions.
   $1-2$ W/cm^2 for $4-5$ minutes (3 MHz for superficial and 1 MHz for deep).
Resorption of exudate.
   Active: $0.25-0.75$ W/cm^2 for $3-5$ minutes (3 MHz).
   Chronic: $0.5-1$ W/cm^2 for $3-5$ minutes (3 MHz).
Wound repair.
   $0.25-0.75$ W/cm^2 for $3-4$ minutes (3 MHz) to periphery.
Haematomas.
   Acute: $0.25-0.5$ W/cm^2 to periphery for $3-5$ minutes (3 MHz).
   Chronic: $0.5-1$ W/cm^2 for $3-5$ minutes.
Resorption of calcium.
   $1.5-3.0$ W/cm^2 for $3-5$ minutes (1 MHz).
NB: The lower the frequency, the better the results.

Great care must be taken with small animals and pulsed settings always used.

8 / Low Powered or Cold Laser Therapy

The lack of success reported by many practitioners trying out cold lasers as a therapeutic agent has, in most cases, been due to a lack of understanding of the equipment and its effects. Lasers are *not* a 'cure-all'.

Light

Light has been used to aid healing since earliest times; *The Rig-Veda*, India's sacred book, allegedly written in 4000 BC, describes the healing power of light. In 1917, Einstein theorized and in 1965 Mestner studied, the biological and physiological effects of low powered lasers on tissue.

Terminology

In order to understand all types of laser (hot and cold) various units of measurement need to be understood.

Nanometer (Na): the unit used to measure the wavelength of light.

Joule (J): the rating for the work (energy) output of a laser (a measurement similar to the W/cm^2 output of the ultrasound machine).

Watts/milliwatts: the power rating. Cold lasers have an average power of $1-2$ mW.

Properties of laser light

Low divergence: the size of the beam stays the same however far the applicator is from the surface at which it is directed.

Monochromicity: the wavelengths within a laser beam are all the same.

Spatial coherence: as all the wavelengths are similar, greater intensity occurs.

Temperal coherence: maximum amplitude is maintained at a constant due to the wavelength arrangement.

High focusability: because of the single wavelength, the intensity can be focused as a very small point.

Collimation: the production of light with similar parallel waves.

Laser light may be visible or invisible; it is created by the bombardment of electrons contained in a specific medium. These electrons tend to remain in a specific orbit; if an energy source is applied to 'push' electrons into a different orbit they will spontaneously return to their original orbit—in so doing they emit light energy. The wavelength created depends upon the electron movement from orbit to orbit. The light source will be amplified by the amount of stimulation or energy applied to push electrons into differing orbits; the greater the stimulus the greater the emission of radiation—**L**ight **A**mplification by **S**timulated **E**mission of **R**adiation (laser).

Cold lasers (therapeutic) (Fig. 8.1)
Helium neon (HeNe)
Historically the first available low powered laser.
The beam is a visible red, delivered at 632.8 nm.
Delivery may be pulsed or continuous.

Gallium arsenide (GaAs) IR
Depending on the wavelength, there may or may not be a visible beam.
Delivery may be pulsed or continuous.

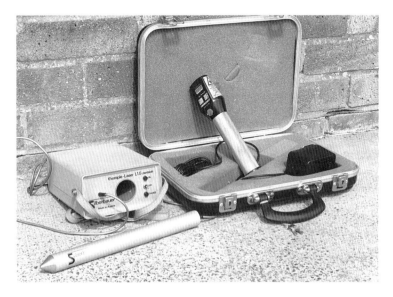

Fig. 8.1 Two battery powered lasers. HeNe on the left and GaAs on the right.

The HeNe and GaAs lasers form the basis of all the presently available products, whose wavelength choices embrace 660, 780, 820 and 904 nm. There is evidence to suggest that the wavelengths of the HeNe laser penetrate approximately 3 mm to 1 cm of tissue thickness and the pulsed GaAs penetrates from 1 to 5 cm of tissue thickness.

Effects of cold laser therapy
Opinions are still divided as to the physiological events that occur at cellular level. The effects can be summarized by stating that the laser beam penetrates into the tissues where it is absorbed by cells and converted into energy, therefore influencing the process of metabolism.

Collagen metabolism. Abergel *et al.* (1984) [21] subjected human skin fibroblasts in culture to exposure using both HeNe and GaAs laser. The results indicated that procollagen production was enhanced by both lasers.

Technique for cold laser therapy (Fig. 9.2)
Soft tissue
Clip and clean the area to be irradiated.
Shield the eyes of the animal and the operator if the manufacturer suggests this.
Conceive a 'grid' of 1-cm squares over the area to be treated, direct the beam at 90° to the centre of each square and focus for approximately 30 seconds.
The probe (or cluster head) should be held just above the body's surface.

Wounds
Clip the hair around the periphery,
Remove dressings, clean the wound.
Treat around the periphery.
Redress the wound (the HeNe laser seems to be the most effective for wound healing).

   If treatment is started within 24 hours 'proud flesh' does not develop and secondary infection is controlled. The wound can then heal without scarring and normal hair growth occurs.

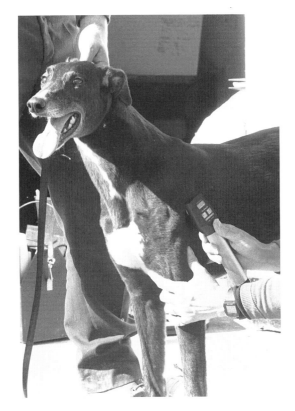

Fig. 8.2 Laser therapy for a tear in the triceps brachii, to reduce pain before muscle stimulation.

The rate of wound healing improves but over-treatment appears to result in the development of collagen lacking in the correct tensile strength and if stressed too early the wound will break down.

Laser acupuncture
There are two major benefits of laser acupuncture.
It is non-invasive.
There is no sensation associated with the beam.
Acupuncture is a science in itself and is not pertinent to this text. GaAs lasers with a reasonable penetration depth have been successfully used by qualified acupuncturists.

INDICATIONS
Pain relief.
Wound healing.
Foot growth. Eustace (Bristol, 1989) [22] has demonstrated that irradiation of the coronary band has marginally improved the rate of growth and texture of the hoof wall.
Neuropraxia. Radial paralysis in the horse, vertebral nerve compressions in small animals have been successfully treated.
Improved recovery for soft tissue trauma has been claimed but work done [23] in Canada suggests the improvement in the first instance is cosmetic and is due to the increased resorption of the inflammatory exudate around the lesion; this is secondary to pain relief and reduction of local spasm.

CONTRAINDICATIONS
Neoplasia.

Dosage levels and treatment times
The wavelength (Na) of the laser chosen determines the dosage and exposure required. The approximate depth of the lesion, the type of lesion and the effects required must all be taken into account. Mester [24] based his calculations for effective biostimulation on a delivery of 4 J/cm^2.
• *Chronic conditions* require higher frequencies and long pulse durations.
• *Acute conditions* require lower frequencies and short pulse durations.

9 / Interferential Therapy

The unit comprises a generator and four sets of pads which may be suction or flat pads (Fig. 9.1). Two medium frequency currents of around 4000 Hz are employed in such a manner that they cross each other and at the meeting point generate a consistent vibration which continues until the machine is switched off. The placement of the four electrodes is as critical as knowing the precise area of the lesion, because the damaged tissue must be contained within the centre of the area at which the two current paths cross. One advantage of interferential therapy is the ability to treat deep seated lesions such as the inferior aspect of the sacro-iliac joint of the horse. A second advantage is that medium frequency currents are able to pass through the skin with a minimum of impedance. Low frequency currents meet a high skin resistance and high frequency currents create a severe thermal reaction; thus neither are suitable for treating deep sited lesions.

The units are usually designed with two oscillators. One circuit

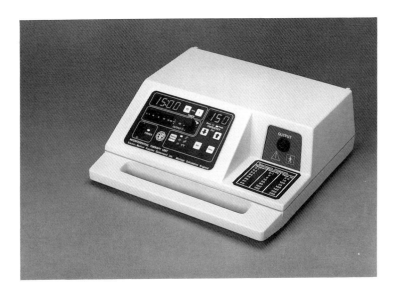

Fig. 9.1 Battery powered interferential unit.

operates at a fixed frequency and the second can be varied; thus the vibration rate or frequency swing can be adjusted to produce a desired result.

Effects on tissue

Pain reduction
Set at 100 Hz constant. The system influences the sensory nerve endings giving an analgesic effect with all its accompanying benefits [25].

Muscle contraction
Set at 1–10 Hz constant. There is a specific effect on motor nerves causing muscle contraction. As the skin allows the passage of the current freely, there is minimal sensory stimulus so that deep sited muscles can be stimulated. Only normally innervated muscle tissue will respond.

Vasodilation
Venous and lymphatic flow increase and the removal of oedema is accelerated with all settings.

Relief of neuralgic type pain
Set at 90–100 Hz rhythmic. The effects are analgesic. In the human, migraine and brachial neuralgia are relieved [26].

Resorption of exudate
Set at 1–10 Hz rhythmic. A stimulating effect to the motor nerve occurs concurrently with a vasodilatory effect. Applied to an area where the exudate is tenacious, there will be improved resorption.

Technique
The coat must be short or clipped under the site for electrode placement. If the machine is powered from the mains use a bib or muzzle (battery machines are available).
Position the unit safely.
Position the patient.
Insulate any skin lesions within the treatment area with vaseline.
Make certain the electrode placement areas are grease-free and any liniments or rubs have been washed out.

Soak the electrode pads in 1% saline solution.

Select frequency: constant or rhythmic.

Test on yourself by placing all four pads on your forearm and turning up the intensity dial.

Turn off machine.

Place electrodes firmly on the appropriate areas making certain the two circuits will cross at the site of the injury.

Position the electrodes so that should two be close to each other, they are of the same polarity. (If they are of different polarity the current will take the path of the least resistance and leak across the space, using the skin as a pathway.)

Turn on the machine.

If the animal is in any way distressed, turn off the unit. The treatment should *not* cause discomfort.

At the end of the treatment time turn down the intensity.

Switch off.

Remove electrodes and inspect the skin.

Wash thoroughly and dry.

Dangers
• Burns can be caused by: (a) bare metal touching the skin; (b) skin currents if electrodes are incorrectly placed; and (c) pads not sufficiently moist.
• Haematoma. If the pressure is too high or the suction speed incorrect, a haematoma may result.

Poor results
• Incorrect choice of frequency for the condition.
• Incorrect circuit balancing.
• Incorrect electrode positioning.

Suitable conditions
• Deep muscle and ligament tears especially in the horse.
• Oedema following trauma or in a joint.
• Haematoma.
• Relief of pain when chemical analgesia is contraindicated.
• Delayed union.

CONTRAINDICATIONS
Infection.

Pregnancy.

Recent injury such as haemarthrosis or where there is danger of
further haemorrhage.

Tumours.

Open wounds.

Dosage

Unfortunately the meter does not register the exact amount of
current passing into the tissues. The reaction of the patient is the
guideline. Choose the setting after deciding the effect required (see
effects on tissue). Treatment is usually given for 10–15 minutes.

The reduction of pain reduces muscle spasm, allows re-establish-
ment of circulatory flow and improves local function in the damaged
tissues. Even if the analgesia is temporary, 10–15 minutes of treatment can produce pain relief of an hour or more. The benefits that
occur in that time are undeniable.

10 / Electrovet and Ionicare

The Ionicare unit was the first electrical stimulator to be designed specifically for animal use. Hard on the heels of the Ionicare came the Electrovet with pads designed in sizes suitable for large and small animal treatment.

The unit output and technique are similar and will be discussed as the same. The type of current delivered is a negative pulsed low frequency current. The pulse/second ratio and intensity are both adjustable for three settings:

1   Leg: 1 pulse/second.
2   'High' muscle: 100 pulses/second.
3   'Low' muscle: 90 pulses/second.

As research into electrotherapy developed and the influence of externally applied currents was explored, it became obvious that ion activity at the cell membrane was increased not by the passage of the current but by the electrical disturbance created.

The main effect of the increased ion activity was to improve the synthesis and activity of potassium—manganese dependent adenosintriphosphatase [27]. This in turn promoted a normal chain reaction of electrochemical changes ending with an increased production of DNA.

It appears that the effects following current application are to stabilize the normal cells and aid the restoration to normal of cells electrically out of balance, due to the hypotoxicity caused by the primary injury. Two pads or electrodes are employed to achieve the desired current effect. A large surcingle contains the anode and a second much smaller pad acts as the cathode. The size of the anode (surcingle) is designed proportionately to allow two cathodes (small pads) to be employed at the same time and still achieve the desired results.

Effects of leg setting

The resorption of an acute palpable oedema in a 'filled' leg or joint, is visibly obvious at the conclusion of treatment. With a 'woody' type chronic 'filling' the combination of ultrasound and Electrovet or Ionicare is beneficial. The area is treated with 3—4 minutes of ultrasound and the Electrovet or Ionicare is applied immediately. It would appear that the claims of the resorption effect of the current stimulus are the most creditable.

Effects of muscle setting
By activating a second circuit, housed in the stimulator, a wave form designed to effect a muscle contraction is produced. Skin sensation appears minimal and with a cathode placed over or near a motor point, stimulation of superficial muscles is achieved. The unit is battery operated and is rechargeable.

General technique (Fig. 10.1)
Position the animal.
Soak the coat beneath the surcingle area.
Soak and partially wring out the towel provided.
Fold to conform to surcingle size.
Place on the body ensuring there are no creases.
Strap surcingle firmly into place.

Technique for leg setting
Soak the skin area over the lesion.
Apply gel.
Bandage or strap electrode (cathode) over the area.
Mount unit on surcingle having tested to see if it is charged.
Attach electrode leads.
Switch on.
Turn up intensity until the animal demonstrates a sensory response, i.e. stamping leg or moving.
Turn back intensity one digit.
Leave for 20–30 minutes.

Techniques for muscle setting
Change switch on unit to 'muscle'. Choose high or low.
Proceed exactly as for 'leg' but soak and gel area over muscle.
Hand hold the pad.
Allow muscle to contract approximately ten times.
Rest 15–20 seconds and repeat.
Treat for up to 20 minutes.

At the conclusion of either treatment turn off unit.
Remove electrodes.

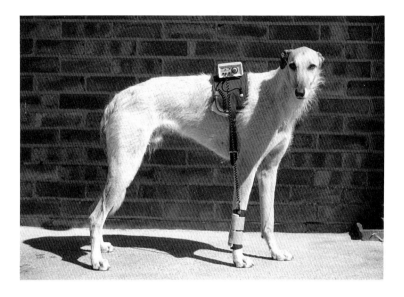

Fig. 10.1 Lurcher being treated with the electrovet for a sprained carpus (wrist).

Wash skin area thoroughly and dry.
Rinse electrodes including towel thoroughly and allow to dry.

INDICATIONS
Leg setting:
   bruising;
   'filled' joints;
   'filled' legs;
   windgalls.
Muscle setting: muscle weakness (all types).

CONTRAINDICATIONS
Infection.
Neoplasia.
Sensory loss.

11 / Rehabilitation

An unnatural way of moving is adopted during the period of injury. The dog or cat may run on three legs avoiding using the injured limb, the horse may shorten its stride or become 'stiff' on one circle and unfortunately, these habits often remain following clinical recovery. The abnormal way of moving has become the cortical imprint or reflex and, for a full recovery, the animal must be 're-educated'. In order to achieve this the animal needs to be placed in a movement sequence, the performance of which will re-establish the correct reflex.

For rehabilitation to be successful, the patient must repeat the correct inbalance movement sequences in a pain-free state to re-establish the correct reflex pattern of movement [28].

Swimming (Figs 11.1 and 11.2)
This is a non-weight-bearing exercise in which the limbs work against the resistance of the water in a symmetrical pattern. When possible use the sea; the extra buoyancy and increased resistance are both of benefit. The animal must swim in straight lines for rehabilitation. If this is not possible, use a heart-rate monitor to determine the stress factor. If animals become exhausted, the anaerobic situation created is detrimental. Horses and dogs inhale deeply as they enter the water, and exhale very little during the swimming session. As they become exhausted and distressed, they inhale in short bursts but do not exhale sufficiently. Most first-time swimmers work anaerobically. The first session should be short; one circuit or once through a straight pool is sufficient. Allow the heart and respiration to return to normal before the second attempt. NB: greyhounds rarely swim well and some cannot swim at all.

Rehabilitation method for horses (Figs 11.3 and 11.4)
The hind shoes should be removed and the horse fitted with good boots, preferably the Clarendon type. Fix a long rope on each side of the noseband of a webbing cavesson; nylon yacht ropes are the best. Put the horse in the entrance pen with an attendant on each side of the head, holding the ropes. First-time swimmers need a rope held behind them by two further attendants. Allow the horse a

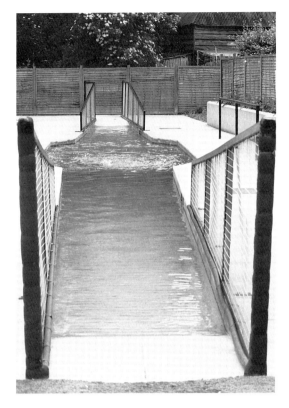

Fig. 11.1 A straight swimming pool. The resistance can be varied by the use of underwater jets.

little time to paw the water and /or sniff it then urge him forward. The attendants with the rear rope may need to use this rope as if they were helping the horse into starting stalls. Once in the water keep the head and neck straight. Do not allow the quarters to drop and swing below the front legs, as this may cause the horse to somersault backwards and drown. The length of time the horse swims must be gauged to his fitness. Scrape off after swimming and dry under a solarium and/or rug up with thermalactic type rugs until the animal is dry.

Rehabilitation method for dogs
Small dogs will usually swim to their owner when lowered into the

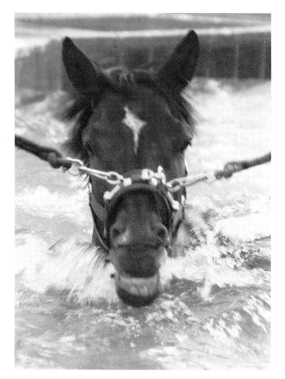

Fig. 11.2 A horse swimming. Note the closed outer nostril. Normal respiration does not occur.

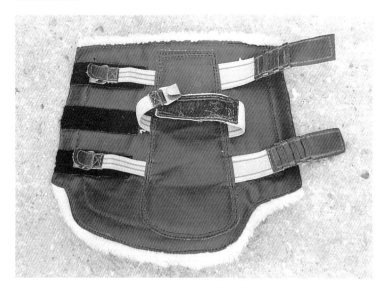

Fig. 11.3 A Clarendon boot; the only make which gives adequate protection to equine swimmers.

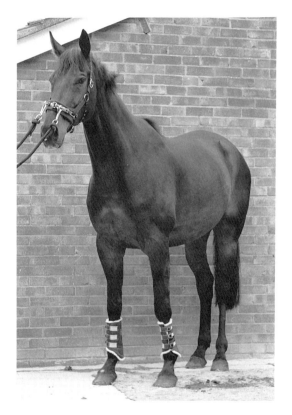

Fig. 11.4 A horse prepared for swimming.

water. Larger dogs should be swum with two attendants, each with a rope to the collar. Scrape off and dry under a solarium if available.

Treadmills (Fig. 11.5a,b)
The moving belt of the treadmill ensures that the animal must move using all four limbs evenly in order to remain in balance; it is excellent for the re-education of the gait pattern in both horses and dogs.

Position of the treadmill
The treadmill should be under cover with a wall facing the moving animal. This prevents distraction and reduces the risk of the thoroughbred racehorse thinking it is a starting stall!

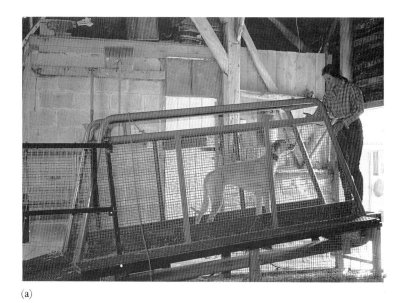

(a)

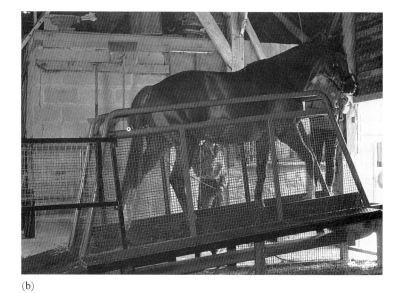

(b)

Fig. 11.5(a,b) A treadmill with a fixed inclination of 6°. Speed up to 6 mph walk.

Types of treadmill
1 A revolving belt, not inclined. Speeds up to a horse's gallop.
2 A revolving belt that can be inclined as the animal works. Speeds up to a horse's gallop.
3 A revolving belt working at a fixed incline (6° is said to be adequate; a greater angulation has been shown to cause hock strain as the animal fatigues). Speeds up to a 6 mph walk.
4 The Equatred. A revolving belt sited on the floor of a water-filled trough. Speeds up to 6 mph walk. This machine is excellent for strengthening the limb and back muscles. Work on a treadmill is very demanding mentally and physically and animals fatigue quickly. Start with 2 minutes and work up over 10 days to 20 minutes.

The walker (Fig. 11.6)
Until recently animals have been tied to the revolving arms of the walker. The latest device allows the animal to be free in an enclosed pen allowing natural balanced movement. The outer pen is 10 metres in diameter and the inner is 7.7 metres giving a pen 2.5 metres by 1.5 metres wide. Start with 5 minutes in each direction

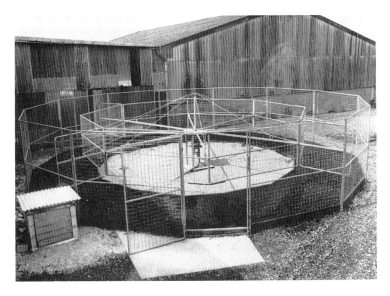

Fig. 11.6 A horse walker with individual pens. The horses work loose, dogs should be tied.

and work up to 20−30 minutes. Dogs may need to be tied for their first sessions. The walker is very useful for greyhounds and all large breeds.

Use of weights (Fig. 11.7)
As previously discussed, muscle wastage follows injury. To re-build and gain the pre-injury state the muscle groups involved need an increased workload which can be achieved by weighting the injured limb.

The dog
- Take a 6 oz strip of lead and bind with masking tape.
- Bend the strip to fix it around the appropriate leg.
- Instruct the owner to use the weight for 10 minute periods during the daily walk (10−21 days).
- This is also an excellent way of persuading a dog or cat to use a previously 'carried' leg.

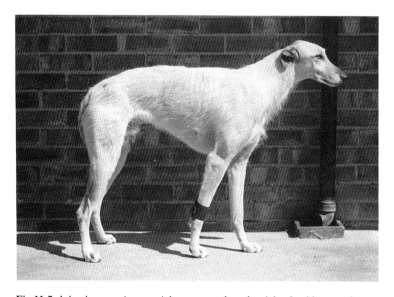

Fig 11.7 A lurcher wearing a weight to strengthen the right shoulder muscles.

The horse
- Purchase an athletic weight 1.5−2 kg from a sports shop, or ask the farries to weight the shoe on the injured limb. To use athletic weight.
- Place a piece of gamgee above the fetlock of the appropriate limb.
- Bandage weight into place with a tail bandage.
- Work the horse for 10−15 minutes twice daily with the weight until the muscle recovers (10−21 days).

The walker creates excellent conditions for working with a weight on a limb.

The aim of rehabilitation is to produce an animal, after treatment, in a physical and mental state which will allow it to return to its previous life-style. The machines alone will not do this. Active exercise, controlled and graduated, must be included within the treatment programme. Owners are usually reasonably co-operative if the reasons for restricted exercise are explained and a programme outlined.

12 / Common Sites of Injury in the Horse and the Dog

The machines aid recovering tissue. There is an unfortunate tendency for owners to expect accelerated recovery and to demand a 'better machine' if immediate miracles are not accomplished. Rather as it is possible to grow prize plants with careful husbandry, so it is possible to put tissue in the best possible situation to allow healing to take place with selective, but restricted, use of physiotherapy machines. Listed in the tables are some of the more common sites and types of injury seen in both horses and dogs.

Conditions in the dog have not been described in such detail as those of the horse, for dogs tend to sustain injuries common to their breed or occupation. The machines or methods suggested have been listed in an order based on the author's experiences. *This does not mean that other combinations may not be equally successful.* No effective treatment is possible without an accurate diagnosis.

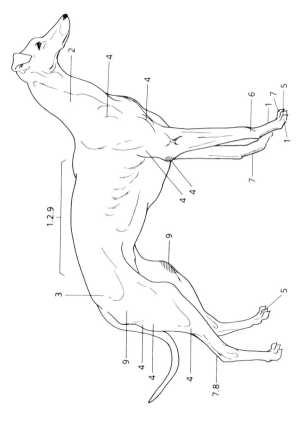

Fig. 12.1 Common sites of injury in the dog.

Table 12.1 Common sites of injury in dogs.

Condition (canine)	Aims of treatment after first aid	Machines appropriate to the condition	Muscles probably involved: stimulate
1 Fractures	Maintain tone in supporting muscles Retain movement in adjacent joints Re-educate after removal of cast	MFT* in cast Ultrasound is contraindicated	Stimulate supporting muscles
2 Neuropraxia	Re-establish nerve conduction Maintain muscle tone	Cold laser at site of compression Massage Passive movements	Stimulate affected muscles
3 Sacro-iliac joint strain		Ultrasound (3 MHz pulsed; 0.25 W/cm^2 × 3 minutes) MFT Deep massage	Stimulate middle gluteal muscles and iliopsoas on injured side
4 Muscle tears	Treat haematoma and stimulate muscles involved	MFT Ultrasound (3 MHz pulsed; 0.25 W/cm^2 × ³⁄₄ minutes) Massage	Stimulate muscles

Table 12.1 Continued.

Condition (canine)	Aims of treatment after first aid	Machines appropriate to the condition	Muscles probably involved: stimulate
5 Web tears	Aid healing	Cold laser	
6 Joint sprains (Carpus very common)	Maintain muscle power Remove inflammation	Ultrasound (3 MHz pulsed; 0.25 W/cm² × 3 minutes) Electrovet Massage	Stimulate all supporting muscles,
7 Tendon tears	Prevent adhesions Maintain muscle power	Cold laser Ultrasound (3 MHz pulsed: 0.25 W/cm² × 3 minutes) Electrovet	Stimulate supporting muscles including parent muscles of tendon involved
8 Tendonitis	Reduce inflammation	Cold Massage: friction Ultrasound (3 MHz pulsed; 0.25 W/cm² × 3–4 minutes)	Stimulate parent muscles of tendons
9 Joint sub-luxation	Improve supporting muscles	MFT Muscle stimulation	Stimulate supporting muscles

10 Ligament tears	Support joint	Cold laser Massage MFT Ultrasound (3 MHz pulsed; 0.25 W/cm^2 × 3–5 minutes)	Stimulate supporting muscles
11 Wounds Road traffic accident or post surgical	Prevent infection Aid healing	Cold laser Ultrasound to haematoma (3 MHz pulsed; 0.25 W/cm^2)	
12 Paraplegia	Re-establish nerve conduction	Cold laser at site of compression Massage Passive movements	Stimulate affected muscles

*MFT = Magnetic Field Therapy.

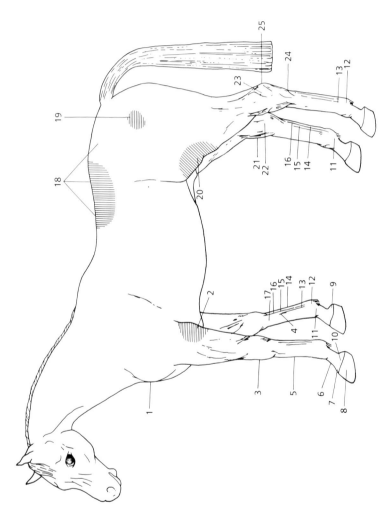

Fig. 12.2 Common sites of injury applicable for physiotherapy treatment in the horse.

Table 12.2 Common sites of injury in horses.

Condition (equine)	Aims of treatment after first aid	Machines appropriate to the condition	Muscles probably involved: stimulate
1 Bicipital bursitis Inflammation of the bursa lying in the bicipital groove near the point of the shoulder	Reduce inflammation Reduce pain Local infiltration with an anti-inflammatory followed by ultrasound is the most effective treatment	Ultrasound (3 MHz 0.25–0.5 W/cm² × 3 minutes)	Deltoid Triceps Pectorals
2 Elbow Capsulitis of the joint following overstretch injury	Establish and remove cause Reduce inflammation Reduce swelling Maintain full range of movement by passive stretching of joint	Ultrasound (3 MHz 0.25–0.5 W/cm² × 3–5 minutes)	Triceps Extensor: carpi radialis Superficial pectoral
3 Knee (a) Direct trauma with bruising and/or lacerations	Reduce swelling Avoid infection Avoid proud flesh Maintain full mobility	Cold between treatments for 3 days Cold laser Ultrasound (3 MHz 0.25 W/cm² × 3 minutes) Passive flexion with fetlock flexed	Deltoid Pectorals Triceps
(b) Capsulitis	Reduce inflammation Maintain full movement	Ultrasound (3 MHz 0.25W/cm² × 3 minutes) Electrovet/Ionicare	

Table 12.2 Continued.

Condition (equine)	Aims of treatment after first aid	Machines appropriate to the condition	Muscles probably involved: stimulate
(c) Surgical removal of bone chips (loose bodies)	Promote healing Avoid adhesions	Laser Massage Passive movements with fetlock flexed *Ultrasound may be contraindicated*	Deltoid Pectorals Triceps
NB: X-ray knee problems			
4 Splint bone (a) Inflammation of the interosseous ligament between the splint and cannon bone. Fusion of the two bones is the end result. Causes: concussion, trauma, uneven shoeing with resultant uneven stress	To promote early fusion with minimal bone formation Maintain fitness	Laser MFT* Swim Ultrasound is contraindicated if a fracture is present. Use with caution	
(b) Fracture of bone may require surgical removal		Laser to incision Check foot balance in all splint cases	
5 Sore shins (a) Inflammation of the periosteum on the front of the cannon bone	Reduce inflammation Promote healing Maintain fitness Reduce concussion	Laser MFT Electrovet/Ionicare Massage with anti-inflammatory cream	Deltoid Triceps Extensor and flexor carpi muscles

(b) Hairline fractures through the front of the cannon bone Causes include concussion, direct trauma, nutritional bone diseases and hind limb problems NB: Sore shins are more common in the fore than hindlimbs. Severe cases may 'buck'. X-ray is advisable to determine severity as all machines have an analgesic effect		MFT *Ultrasound is contraindicated* Swim Specialist pads: EZ Strider or Sorbothane to reduce concussion Check for hind limb lameness and foot balance in forelimb
6 High ringbone	Reduce inflammation Minimize new bone growth Reduce concussion	The value of machine therapy is debatable in all cases of ringbone Try ultrasound (3 MHz 1.0–2.0 $\text{W/cm}^2 \times 3$ minutes)
7 Low ringbone		MFT Swim Specialist pads: EZ Strider or Sorbothane
8 Sandcrack	Promote healthy hoof growth Specialist shoeing to support crack	Laser to coronary band
9 Over reach	Prevent infection Promote healing	Laser Ultrasound (3 MHz 0.25 $\text{W/cm}^2 \times 3$ minutes)

Table 12.2 Continued.

Condition (equine)	Aims of treatment after first aid	Machines appropriate to the condition	Muscles probably involved: stimulate
10 Sidebones	Promote healing with minimal bone formation	Ultrasound (3 MHz 1.0–2.0 W/cm^2 × 3 minutes) MFT	
11 Fetlock joint (ankle) (a) Capsulitis due to sprain	Reduce inflammation Maintain full movement	Cold Ultrasound (3 MHz 0.25–0.5 W/cm^2 × 5 minutes) Electrovet/Ionicare MFT Massage Passive stretching Swim	Deltoid Triceps Pectorals
(b) Bruising due to direct trauma	Reduce bruising	As above	
(c) Degenerative arthritis in older horses	Improve the integrity of the joint capsules	Ultrasound (3 MHz 0.5 W/cm^2 5 minutes) MFT Passive stretching Swim	
(d) Fractures of the pastern or lower end of the cannon may involve the joint	Promote healing	MFT *if not pinned* Massage shoulder and bulbs of heels *Ultra sound is contraindicated*	Forearm muscles

12 Sesamoid bones

(a) Inflammation of one or both of the sesamoids. Often concurrent with problems in the fetlock joint	Reduce inflammation and increase circulatory flow. Maintain full movement. Maintain fitness in acute stage	Laser. Ultrasound (3 MHz 1.0–1.5 W/cm² × 3 minutes). MFT. Electrovet/Ionicare. Massage. Passive stretching. Swim	
(b) Fracture of one or both of the proximal sesamoids. NB: X-ray is advisable in all suspected sesamoid cases	Promote healing	MFT	

13 Windgalls (windpuffs)
There is a distension of the synovial sheath between either the suspensory ligament and cannon bone or between the long pastern and ligament joining the sesamoids

Cause: Overstress of the limb, concussion or incorrect angulation of joints of the foot and pastern

NB: Tends to be more common in the hind than forelegs

Reduce inflammation before the condition becomes chronic. Find and remove cause if possible	Ultrasound (3 MHz 0.25–0.5 W/cm² × 3–5 minutes). Electrovet/Ionicare. Swim	Check for muscle weakness, stimulate weak muscle groups

Table 12.2 Continued.

Condition (equine)	Aims of treatment after first aid	Machines appropriate to the condition	Muscles probably involved: stimulate
14 and 15 Flexor tendons and/or suspensory ligament The superficial, the deep or both may be involved. Partial or complete rupture may occur. Bowing may be present In all cases support of the fetlock joint is reduced. Severe case may be supported by casting	Support the area Reduce swelling Reduce inflammation Promote healing Maintain muscle strength in shoulder or quarter	Compression and cold, i.e. Bonner type bandage followed with Tube Grip Ultrasound(3 MHz 0.25–1.0 W/cm^2 × 3–5 minutes) Electrovet/Ionicare Massage Laser with Electrovet/Ionicare and massage MFT with Electrovet/Ionicare and massage MFT will penetrate a cast. No other machine will be of use if a cast is used	*Forelimb* Deltoid Triceps Pectorals Supraspinatus Infraspinatus Extensor carpi muscles *Hindlimb* Gluteals Hamstrings Quadriceps
16 Check ligament Damage can occur in association with tendon and/ or suspensory injuries or as a separate issue	Reduce inflammation Promote healing Maintain fitness	Treat as for tendons	Stimulate as for tendons
17 Speedy cut Cuts caused by striking one leg with shoe or hoof of another leg	Prevent infection Promote healing	Laser Ultrasound (3 MHz 0.25–0.75 W/cm^2 × 3–5 minutes) MFT	

18 Thoraco-lumbar and/or pelvic problems Opinions vary widely as to the reasons for damage in the spine and pelvis. The problems are thought to be ligament tears with associated muscle weakness. Fractures (hairline cracks in particular) have been observed in many bone specimens along with arthritic and other bony changes	Reduce pain Re-educate muscles Re-educate movement with weight off the back	Ultrasound (1 MHz 0.75–1.0 W/cm^2 for 3–5 minutes) MFT Interferential Deep massage Swim	Longissimus Gluteal
19 Trochanteric bursitis The bursa lies under the tendon of the middle gluteal muscle and above the greater trochanter of the femur. Pressure caused by the contraction of the gluteals compresses the bursa giving rise to shortening of stride and on occasions severe lameness	Reduce inflammation Maintain muscle strength Re-educate movement after reduction of pain	Ultrasound (1 MHz 1.00–2.50 W/cm^2 for 3–5 minutes) MFT Interferential Deep massage Muscle stimulation after reduction of pain Swim	Gluteal muscles Semimembranosus Semitendinosus Biceps femoris

Table 12.2 Continued.

Condition (equine)	Aims of treatment after first aid	Machines appropriate to the condition	Muscles probably involved: stimulate
20 Stifle joint Most stifle problems result from the patella deviating from its normal anatomical position. These movements may cause the joint to 'lock'. Any dislocation of the patella causes extensive ligament stretching and associated muscle weakness	Reduce inflammation if present Strengthen weak muscle groups	Laser Muscle stimulation Massage	Examine for weak muscle groups and stimulate
21 and 22 Spavin (a) Bog spavin. Capsulitis of the hock. The result of stress and or poor conformation	Reduce inflammation	Laser Electrovet/Ionicare Massage in all cases MFT	
(b) Bone spavin: unwanted bone forms usually on the inner surface of the hock interfering with articulation of the joint, or there is erosion of the articular surfaces followed by new bone growth	Reduce inflammation Maintain joint range	(Raise heels of back shoes) Laser or Electrovet/Ionicare Massage in all cases *Ultrasound is contraindicated*	

NB: *In the author's experience the hock is the most unpredictable joint to treat. Treat all cases whatever the condition with great caution*

23 Thoroughpin A swelling of the sheath of the deep flexor tendon of the hock due to trauma or strain	Reduce swelling	Electrovet/Ionicare Ultrasound (3 MHz 0.25 W/cm² × 3 minutes) MFT Massage in all cases Passive movements	Hamstrings
24 Curb Thickening of the plantar tarsal ligament usually caused by over exertion. Poor conformation is a contributory factor	Reduce inflammation Control swelling	Laser and Ultrasound (3 MHz 0.75 W/cm² × 3 minutes) MFT Electrovet/Ionicare Massage in all cases Swim	
25 Capped hock Swelling of the bursa over the point of the hock usually caused by trauma or sitting against the box wall	Reduce inflammation	Cold (Bonner type bandage) Ultrasound (3 MHz 0.5 W/cm² × 3 minutes) Electrovet/Ionicare	

Table 12.2 Continued.

Condition (equine)	Aims of treatment after first aid	Machines appropriate to the condition	Muscles probably involved: stimulate
26 Bruised or torn muscles If left untreated bruising in a muscle will 'scar', i.e. a dense area of fibrous tissue with no elastic properties will form. This will reduce the efficiency of surrounding muscle tissue and when the muscle is at full stretch the tissue above and below the scar will be over stressed and in its turn, tear	Reduce the bruise (haematoma) Maintain maximal muscle efficiency Prevent adhesions	Cold Laser Ultrasound. Dose according to depth and severity of injury MFT Electrovet/Ionicare Massage Controlled exercise	Stimulate immediately

*MFT = Magnetic Field Therapy.

Appendix 1/General Guidelines

Machine therapy, unlike chemotherapy, had no set prescription stating the exact dosage level, treatment time or number of treatments required to 'cure' or 'relieve' a condition. Each case will vary slighty and the suggestions in this text should only be used as guidelines. Where possible, dangerous or ineffective treatment methods have been stated.

It is essential for the person operating a therapy unit to understand the effects of the unit as fully as possible. The type of tissue and the type of lesion to be influenced should be recognized. The machine most effective for that lesion should be chosen and care taken not to over treat.

The literature accompanying most therapy units has been compiled by the manufacturer. Unfortunately not all the information offered in these texts is backed by laboratory proof. Experience is needed to achieve the best results. Physiotherapy has not been recognized as an established veterinary procedure long enough for sufficient clinical records to have been kept and the findings published, but the majority of research has been carried out using laboratory rats and mice.

The effects of one machine may overlap those of another. In order to make the best choice the following questions should be asked.

1 What is the nature of the lesion?
2 Is the problem acute, sub-acute or chronic?
3 Is the site of the lesion superficial or deep?
4 Is the damage localized or has it become diffuse?
5 What pathophysiological changes have occurred?
6 Is the condition going to benefit from machine therapy?
   If so do you require:
   an analgesic effect?
   a thermal effect?
   a massage effect?
   resorption effects?
7 What type of structure do you wish to influence?
   Bone?
   Joint: capsule or ligaments?
   Tendon?
   Muscle?
   Nerve?
   Blood vessels?
   Lymphatic vessels?
Having considered the nature of the lesion, the effects required and the tissue type, a constructive choice of therapy can be achieved.

All the guidelines assume skin sensation is normal and the nerve supply intact.

Cold

Water wellies
Hosing   20 minutes 3–4 times a day.

Cold bandages
Ice   20 minutes every 2 hours in acute phase, up to 70 hours.

Cold laser

30/90 seconds to each point of an imagined 1 cm² grid. Treat on alternate days for up to 10 days; if recovery is not complete, rest for a week and repeat.

NB: Most manufacturer's literature suggests treatment programmes. Many of these programmes have a cosmetic result, tissue appearing to have recovered. In many cases the tensile strength of the tissue is inadequate and there is a danger of breakdown, *so resume activity with caution.* Lasers should only be used by qualified personnel.

Electrovet

Leg setting. Adjust to patient's tolerance. Treat for up to one hour daily, overtreating may blister. Treat for up to 10 days.

Muscle setting. Treat muscle for up to 20 minutes twice daily. Three weeks treatment should be sufficient; only superficial muscle groups appear to be influenced.

Heat

Acute lesions. Low intensity for 20–30 minutes twice daily.

Chronic lesions. Heat to tolerance without causing a burn. 15–20 minutes twice daily. As the condition improves try to treat *before* exercise.

Interferential

Adjust the settings for patient comfort. It is *essential* to position the electrodes in a manner that ensures that the lesion lies in the centre of the cross-over paths of the two currents. If this does not occur the treatment will be ineffective.

This machine should only be used by an experienced operator.

Massage
Treat for 10–15 minutes twice daily in acute stage of injury.
Treat for 10–15 minutes daily in chronic stage of injury.

Magnetic field therapy
Treat according to instruction manual. Animals may resent MFT. This
may indicate the setting chosen is incorrect and is causing pain or the
diagnosis is incorrect. Animals presenting with back pain diagnosed as
'muscular' exhibit discomfort if the back ache is the result of a problem in
the kidneys.

Muscle stimulators

Faradic type. 15–20 minutes daily.

Trophic stimulators. Start with 15 minutes and work up to 1 hour daily.
Three weeks treatment should effect recovery. Damage to the motor nerve
requires daily treatment until conduction returns.

Ultrasound
Treat for 3–5 minutes according to the type of lesion.
This machine should only be used by experienced operators.

Appendix 2/Suppliers of Machines Suitable for Animal Physiotherapy

General suppliers

Australia

TES Electronic Pyt Ltd, Unit 6, 5 Ladd Road, Gisborneshire Industrial Estate, New Gisborne, Victoria 3438

Canada

Fetouris Int Ltd, 9674 Street, NR3 Delta DC, British Columbia, Canada.

UK

Animal Therapy Ltd, Tyringham Hall, Cuddington, Aylesbury, Buckinghamshire HP18 0AS.

Medipost Ltd, 100 Shaw Road, Oldham OL1 4AY

USA

Fetouris Int Ltd, 256 North Highway, 101 Encinitas, San Diego, California, 92024.

Cold sources

Bonner Bandage: Equetech Ltd, 18 Shawfield Street, London SW3 4BD.

Wellie Boots: Animal Therapy Ltd, Tyringham Hall, Cuddington, Aylesbury, Buckinghamshire HP18 0AS.

Jacuzzi Tub: Newmarket Requisites, Black Bear Lane, Newmarket, Suffolk CB8 0JT

Thermacold Legwrap: Equine Innovation, c/o PO Box 1209, Wildomar, California 923915.

Cold laser

Electro Medical Supplies (Wantage) Ltd, Wantage, Oxon OX1 7AD.

Electrovet

Electrovet Ltd, 3 Reading House, Henley-on-Thames, Oxon RG9 1AB.

Equine pool

Rainbow Pools, Ocean House, Beachmore Road, London SW11 4ET.

All Seasons Leisure, 1 Edison Road, Churchfields, Salisbury, Wilts SP2 7NU

Heat sources

Chaud Cheval: 8 Cobden Avenue, Mexborough, South Yorkshire S64 0AD.

Equine Thermaskin: Vulkan UK Ltd, 11 Newarke Street, Leicester LE1 5SS

Newmarket Requisites, Black Bear Lane, Newmarket, Suffolk CB8 0JT

Sunlight

Solarium: Newmarket Requisites, Black Bear Lane, Newmarket, Suffolk
   CB8   0JT.
Hippolarium: Alvescot International Ltd, 2 Bollin Tower, Alderley Edge, Cheshire
   SK9   7BY.

Horse walker

John Funell, Ash Tree Farm, Staverton, Daventry, Northants NN11   4NN.

Interferential units

Electro Medical Supplies (Wantage) Ltd, Wantage, Oxon OX12   7AD.

Magnetic field therapy

Animal Therapy Ltd, Tyringham Hall, Cuddington, Aylesbury, Buckinghamshire
   HP18   0AS.
MH Electronics Ltd, 13 Western Road, Wolverton, Milton Keynes, Buckingham-
   shire MK12   5AY.

Magnetic pads

EPC, 1 Friggle Street, Frome Somerset BA11   5LH.

Muscle stimulators

Faradic (battery operated)
Electro Medical Supplies (Wantage) Ltd, Wantage, Oxon OX12   7AD.

Orthotron & neuromuscular stimulator
Raymar, PO Box 16, Fairview Estate, Reading Road, Henley-on-Thames, Oxon
   RG9   1LL.

Massage machines

Niagara Therapy (UK) Ltd, Colomerdy Industrial Estate, Rhyl Road, Denbeigh,
   North Wales.
Pifco: Any branch of Boots the Chemists; John Bell and Croydon, Wigmore Street,
   London WIM   7DE.

Treadmill and Equatred

Pegasus Exerciser: Sportsfield Machines Ltd, Athena House, London Road, Morden
   SM4   5AZ.

Ultrasound machines

Electro Medical Supplies (Wantage) Ltd, Wantage, Oxon OX12   7AD.

References

1 Wyke BD. (1981) Neurological aspects of pain therapy. A review of current concepts. In: Swerdlow M. (ed.) *The Therapy of Pain. (Current status of modern therapy)* 1st edn. Chap 1, pp. 1-30. MTP Press Ltd, Lancaster.

2 Salter RB, Harris DJ. (1979) The healing of intra-articular fractures with continuous passive motion. *Am Acad Orthop Surg* Lecture Series 6: **28**, 102-117

3 Salter RB. Regeneration of articular cartilage through continuous passive motion. In: *Clinical Trends in Othopoedics*.

4 Wadsworth H, Chanmugan APP. (1988) Physiological effects of heat and cold. In: *Electrophysical Agents in Physiotherapy* 2nd edn. Science Press, Marrickville. Downey JA. (1964) Physiological effects of heat and cold. *Phys Therm.* **44**(8): 713-717

5 Murphy AJ. (1960) Physiological effects of cold application. *Phys Ther Rev* **40**: 122-115

6 Lewis T, Hagnal I, Kerr W, Stern E. (1930) Observations upon the reaction of human tissue to cold and heat. *Am J Med Sci* **15**: 177-208

7 Warnke V. (1980) Magnetomedicines. In: *Verlagsegellschaft fur Biophysik und Medizin*. Proceedings of 2nd International Symposium on Magnetic Field Medicine. Rome

8 Melzack R, Wall PD. (1965) Pain mechanisms: a new theory. *Science* 150: 971-979

9 Watson J, Downes EM. (1979) Clinical aspects of the stimulation of bone healing using electrical phenomena. *Med Biol Eng Comput* **17**: 161-169

10 Salter RB, Hamilton HW, Wedge JH, Tile M, Torode IP, O'Driscoll SW, Murnaghann JJ, Saringer JH. (1984) . . . . . The clinical application of basic research on continuous passive motion for disorders and injuries of synovial joints. *J Orthop Res* **1**(3), 325-342

11 Cooper AP. (1965) On dislocation of the ankle joint. In: De Palma AF (ed.) *Clin Orthop Rel Res* **42** (part 1): 2
Clayton ML, Weir GJ. (1959) Experimental investigations of ligamentous healing. *Am J Surg* 98: 373-378

12 O'Donovan MJ. (1985) Developmental regulations of motor function. *Med Sci Sports Exerc* 17(1): 35-43
Vrbova G, Navarrete, Lowrie M. (1985) Matching of muscle properties and motor-neurone firing patterns. *J Exp Biol* 15: 133-123

13 Scott O, Vrbova G, Dubowitz W. (1984) Effects of nerve stimulation on normal and diseases muscle. Raven Press, New York

14 Farragher DJ, Kidd GL, Tallis R. (1987) Rational of cotrophic stimulation. *Clin Rehab* 1: 265-271

15 Melzack R, Wall D. (1988) In: *The Challenge of Pain*. 2nd edn. MTP Press Ltd, Lancaster

16 Dyson M, Pond JB. (1970) The effects of pulsed ultrasound on tissue regeneration. *Physiotherapy* 56: 136-142

17 Wadsworth H, Chanmugan APP. (1988) In: *Electrophysical Agents in Physiotherapy* 2 edn, p. 122. Science Press, Marrickville

18 Wadsworth H, Chanmugan APP. (1988) *Electrophysical Agents in Physiotherapy* 2 edn, p. 123. Science Press, Marrickville

19 Griffin JE. (1966) Physiological effects of ultrasonic energy as it is used clinically. *J Am Phys Ther* 46: 18-26

20 Wadsworth H, Chanmugan APP. (1988) In: *Electrophysical Agents in Physiotherapy* 2 edn, p. 126. Science Press, Marrickville

21 Abergel RP, Meeker CA, Dwyer RM, Le Savoy MA, Vitto J. (1984) Non-thermal effects of the Nd: YAG laser on biological functions of human skin fibroblasts in culture. *Laser Surg Med* 3: 279-284

22 Eustace R. (1989) Irradiation of the coronary band with a GaAs laser. (Pers Commun) Bristol.

23 McKibbin LS. (1988) Low level laser therapy in veterinary practice on standard bred horses. In: Ohshiro T, Calderhead RG (eds) *Low Level Laser Therapy* pp. 77-80. John Wiley & Son, Chichester

24 Mester E, Mester A. (1985) The biomedical effects of laser application *Laser Surg. Med* 5: 31-39

25 Deller AGM. (1984) Physical principles of interferential therapy. In: Savage B (ed) *Interferential Therapy* Chap 1, pp. 17-26. Faber & Faber, London

26 Savage B (ed.) (1987) *Interferential Therapy* Chap 6, pp. 69-73. Faber & Faber, London

27 Vasko KA. (1986) The equine athlete. In: *Progress in Equine Therapy* pp. 9-11, Ohio

28 Astrand P-O, Rodahl K. (eds) (1970) *Textbook of Work Physiology* 2 edn. McGraw-Hill, New York
Langleyl L, Telford IR, Christenson RB. (1974) *Dynamic Anatomy and Physiology* McGraw-Hill, New York
Mathews DK, Fox EL. (1976) *The Physiological Basis of Physical Education and Athletics.* WB Saunders, Philadelphia
Basmajian JV. (1979) *Muscles Alive* 4th edn. Williams & Wilkins, Baltimore
Janda V (1976) Muskel functions diagnostic. Student Litteratur. Lund
Astrand P-O, Rodahl K. (eds). (1977) *Textbook of Work Physiology* 2 edn. McGraw-Hill, New York
O'Donoghue. (1976) Treatment of injuries to athletes. In: *Rehabilitation.* pp. 791-821. WB Saunders, Philadelphia

Index